Finding
BALANCE

Empower Yourself with Tools

To Combat Stress and Illness—So You Can

Live A Longer, Healthier Life

MONICA AGGARWAL, MD

JYOTHI RAO, MD

Colleen
Be empowered to
change!
John, MD

Finding
BALANCE

Empower Yourself with Tools
To Combat Stress and Illness—So You Can
Live A Longer, Healthier Life

Prescriptions for a Better, More Vital You

MONICA AGGARWAL, MD

JYOTHI RAO, MD

TWO MINDS PRESS
Clarksville Maryland

Finding BALANCE
Empower Yourself with Tools to Combat Stress and Illness—
So You Can Live a Longer, Healthier Life
by Monica Aggarwal, MD & Jyothi Rao, MD

Designed by Robert L. Lascaro
www.lascarodesign.com
Typeset in ITF Stone Serif and Helvetica Neue

Printed in the United States
Printer: Lightning Source

ISBN: 978-0-692-47603-1

Published by
Two Minds Press,
Clarksville MD 21029

Contact:
Monica Aggarwal, MD
www.drmonicaaggarwal.com

Jyothi Rao, MD
www.raowellness.com

EDITOR'S NOTE:
This book contains the opinions and general thoughts of the authors. The prescriptions in the book are meant only as general guidelines. The book is by no means intended as a substitute for the medical advice of your personal physicians. The reader should regularly consult a physician in matters relating to his/her health or need for any advice related to exercise, diet, role of yoga, sleep, personal health or any other assistance. Specifically, a qualified physician should be consulted with respect to any symptoms that may require diagnosis or medical attention. The authors, editors, and publisher accept no liability for any injury arising out of the use of material contained herein, and make no warranty, express or implied, with respect to the contents of this publication.

DEDICATION

I dedicate this book to my parents who raised me, my siblings who support me and to my husband who is my light. He has helped me thrive with his calm, his warmth and his love...and to Kai, Maya and Asha who deal with my crazy as the true warriors that they are.

— Monica Aggarwal MD

I dedicate this book to my husband Par and my kids Anjali, Shalin and Kiren for supporting me through this journey...and to my late maternal grandfather Dhruva Rao who inspired me to heal others

— Jyothi Rao MD

CONTENTS

FOREWORD:
Traveling the world researching alternative healing practices
by Andrew Weil, MD **9**

INTRODUCTION: Are You on Fire?
As youth, we have a perception of invincibility and how the choices
we make can overwhelm our body's natural defenses. **11**

1: BALANCE AND HOMEOSTASIS
Balance must occur between resources and demands. When demands
outweigh resources, illness is triggered—the body becomes inflamed: . . **15**

2 HOW MY DAUGHTER SAVED ME:
Dr. Monica Aggarwal's Story

Dr. Aggarwal developed a significant illness that became her defining
life moment and turning point **21**

3 LEARNING THE MEANING OF MD:
Dr. Jyothi Rao's Story

Dr. Rao struggled as a physician not treating patients but illnesses leading
to to her transformative decision to move into a wellness practice . . . **25**

**4 BREAKING DOWN: When balance is disrupted,
stress and inflammation are created**
A detailed look at how chronic illness affects the immune system
and activates the sympathetic nervous system. **29**

5 CHRONIC ILLNESS IS BORN
A detailed look at specific illnesses such as cancer, Diabetes, high
cholesterol and heart disease and how they affect our bodies. **39**

6 THE HOUSE OF BUGS: Learn About Our Gut
The microorganisms in our gut make up our second immune system.
The type of gut bugs we have determine how healthy we are **49**

7 HEAL THY GUT
The elimination diet: removing toxins from our body allows the gut
to heal and perform as a stronger line of defense against illness . . . **71**

8   SUPER FOODS: Greens, Beans, Carbs, Oh My!
A detailed look at the phytonutrients in foods which help
fuel the microbiome and help with lowering inflammation **91**

9   OIL CHANGE: Nuts, Seeds, Avocado and
a conversation about oil
Nuts, seeds, avocado and a conversation about oil—the controversy
over the benefits of oil in different foods sources **107**

10 SPICE IT UP!
Spices offer unique ingredients to help lower inflammation and
oxidative stress. Turn your kitchen cabinets into a medicinal cabinet. . **123**

11 WATER, The Essence Of Life
Water, the essence of life – Learn about the substance which
has the ability to rejuvenate, invigorate and sustain balance. **131**

12 SLEEP ON IT, catching some ZZZZs
Recharge the body to bring back balance from the stresses. Restorative
sleep helps with metabolism, hormone balance, and detoxification . . . **135**

13 THE MIND-BODY CONNECTION
A look at the interplay between the mind and the body. How postures,
breathing techniques and meditation can induce healing. **151**

14 THE EUPHORIA OF EXERCISE
Physical movement sustains balance, protects the heart and
can help with energy, hormone balance and mood. **171**

15 RECHARGE
Recharge: Summary of tools to help rest and digest and bring
back homeostasis **203**

※ ENDNOTES **205**

※ GLOSSARY **229**

※ ACKNOWLEDGMENTS **244**

※ ABOUT THE AUTHOR **245**

Foreword

FindIng new tools to heal the whole body

Andrew Weil, M.D.

WE LIVE IN A WORLD that relies heavily on conventional medicine and, especially, pharmaceutical drugs to manage disease conditions. For acute and critical problems these approaches have tremendous value, but they are less useful in cases of chronic illness, many of which result from unhealthy lifestyle choices. I have been researching alternative healing practices for more than 40 years. After completing my training in conventional medicine, I traveled the world, living with and acquiring knowledge from people of many different cultures. Most of the healing systems I have studied emphasize the role of food choices, sleep, along with natural remedies, mind/body techniques, and spiritual practices to maintain and restore health. Combining some of these ideas and methods with conventional medicine has been the foundation of the integrative medicine that I teach and practice.

FINDING BALANCE IS AN ENGAGING BOOK that recounts the parallel journeys of two skilled physicians, Dr. Monica Aggarwal and Dr. Jyothi Rao, who were motivated to find new tools that would enable them to heal the whole body, not just treat symptoms. I first met Dr. Aggarwal, an energetic and accomplished cardiologist, in 2005. She had a thriving practice, with a commitment to provide the best care for her patients but she was already aware of the limitations of pharmaceuticals and curious about alternative therapies. When she was diagnosed with rheumatoid arthritis in 2011, her search for other ways to treat began in earnest. Dr. Aggarwal offers a frank discussion of her debilitating disease and her path to healing. I am impressed by her transformation and evolution as a physician and how she has learned to incorporate her discoveries into caring for her patients. The positive outcome she experienced is an inspiring testament to the power of choice and control we have in matters of health.

DR. JYOTHI RAO IS A DEDICATED internist who has long held the belief that healing the body involves much more than pills. More and more providers are struggling with the same frustration with conventional medicine that she felt. It led her to pursue acupuncture and functional medicine to help her patients. I admire her relentless effort to create an integrative internal medicine practice that is demonstrating how non-pharmacologic modalities can change lives.

THE BOOK THESE TWO DOCTORS have written is a useful resource for anyone interested in attaining better health. The authors explain how both lifestyle choices and environmental triggers can cause breakdowns in various body systems, and they offer prescriptions with detailed practical tips to correct them. Anyone can make use of this advice to have lasting benefits with only positive side effects. Drs. Aggarwal and Rao draw on available scientific data to support their points and are not afraid to say when data are lacking.

WE KNOW THAT OUR HEALTH is not predetermined by genes alone. It is our day- to-day choices of how we live, environmental influences, stressors and how we handle them that determine health outcomes. The experience of illness is not the same for everyone with the same diagnosis. Treatment must be individualized – there is no one size that fits all. And the impact of lifestyle changes will also differ from person. But I believe the information and tools that Drs. Aggarwal and Rao present in these pages are applicable to all of us and can serve as a guide to achieving optimum health.

Andrew Weil, M.D.

INTRODUCTION

Body on Fire

WE HAVE ONE BODY. We have one life. Everything we do to it from our birth to our old age has an impact. When we are young, we believe we are invincible. We feel we can stress our bodies and they will endure. And they will at the beginning. That is why we keep doing the things we do because we often don't feel the impact until years later. The body is prepared for acute stress. We have stress hormones and systems in place that allow us to deal with acute stress. Our senses become activated and we are more keenly aware of our surroundings. Our immune system is revved up and we are able to deal with insults. But at some point, with more continuous stress, our demand outweighs our resources. Our bodies have only so much reserve and ultimately, our bodies become imbalanced. These stresses come from many external sources such as excess sunlight, pollution, lack of sleep, social and job stress as well as lack of activity. Stress also comes from the foods we ingest such as processed foods, meat and dairy.

When the body becomes imbalanced, it becomes irritated and inflamed. We call that *body on fire*. The body becomes so revved up that the insides become unhappy. The immune system goes into overdrive and switches from a controlled system into a wild, overcharged system that can start hurting itself. It can start attacking its own organs. This inflammation over time ultimately leads to illness. Inflammation manifests differently in everyone. Some people have stomach complaints:

constipation, abdominal pain and diarrhea. Some people experience excessive fatigue, weight gain and depression. Others develop autoimmune disease such as multiple sclerosis, rheumatoid arthritis and inflammatory bowel disease. Still others develop cancer and heart disease. Initially, when we don't feel right, we consult our physicians who see little wrong in the baseline lab results. In further testing, certain markers of inflammation might be elevated but not always at the beginning. These normal test results can leave us feeling unsatisfied and give a false sense of security. Ultimately, we end up ignoring signs or they are too nonspecific for doctors to pinpoint the diagnosis. Then, we develop sickness and are surprised how it happened. We, the authors know, because it has happened to us.

We are all affected in some way or another. It always takes a toll. It is for this reason that we, Dr. Aggarwal (a cardiologist) and Dr. Rao (an internist) have decided to write this book. We have been sick. We know what it feels like to be blindsided by illness yet the signs were there all along. We just weren't looking. As physicians, we started to look for answers first in our pills. When the pills left us with nasty side effects and incomplete healing, we started on a journey to understand why the body gets sick and what we can do to heal it—truly heal it. Over the years, we have learned together that there is so much we can do to put our bodies back in balance. There are so many options for treatments, beyond our pills, to heal our bodies and decrease our inflammation. We have written this book to educate you, offer you hope for options for healing and to empower you with the knowledge and tools to identify your fires and extinguish them.

Healing is not a simple task..but it is a worthwhile one. As physicians, we stand by the medicines that we prescribe but we offer here additional prescriptions that don't come in pill form. These are prescriptions that complement our medications and sometimes, if we are lucky, allow us to stop taking our pills. It happened for us and it happens for so many of our patients. Here in these chapters, we have given you a comprehensive and detailed study and present as much data as is available on these matters. The reality, however, is that much of the data out there is not the desired randomized control trial. There are few studies that will compare diet with pills because of the worry of withholding therapy as well as the significant lack of funding. Often studies are funded by pharmaceutical companies. Pharmaceutical companies want trials because if there are positive associations between illness and the medication, we physicians will prescribe that medication and they will make more money. The problem is that the prescriptions in this book aren't pills. Companies have no incentives to offer solutions that don't include drugs.

Therefore, we present as much data as we could find and as many anecdotes as we can, and you can make your own judgments. You should consider, though, how little you have to lose by trying these prescriptions and how much you could possibly gain. We are not prescribing dangerous changes. You will suffer no medication side effects if you follow our advice. What do you have to lose by trying? These prescriptions changed our lives by extinguishing our fires. We hope they will change yours, too. We want you to be empowered to change—to heal—to balance. Come with us on this journey. Welcome to the new and healthier you!

As you read through this book, we ask you to consider how you feel.

See Table 1 where we have listed questions for you to ask yourself. If you have answered yes to any of these questions, we hope you will take the time to read this book. We also mention baseline testing that we check to assess a person's inflammatory burden and subsequent risk for illness. **Table 2** shows some of the baseline tests.

TABLE 1. HOW DO I FEEL?

ENERGY:

✓ **Do I feel I have energy** to do the things I want to do daily?

✓ **Do I feel rested** when I wake up in the morning?

✓ **Do I feel as if I need a nap** during the day? Such as, right after lunch?

✓ **Am I in pain** when I wake up, or feel pain throughout the day?

LIFESTYLE:

✓ **Am I exercising?** How do I get stronger?

✓ **Am I frustrated with my weight?**

✓ **I want to take fewer pills**, or possibly none at all—which ones can I stop taking?

✓ **Do I sleep enough?**

FOOD:

✓ **How do I feel after eating my food?** Do I get tired? Does my pain get worse?

✓ **Are my meals healthy?** What does that look like? Does my food come in a frozen box? Do I cook or mainly microwave?

✓ **I really don't eat anything but I continue to gain weight?** Why am I always constipated? Do I go to the bathroom every day?

✓ **I crave sweets all of the time.** Is this normal?

MIND:

✓ **I had bad habits my whole life.** Is it too late to change?

✓ **Do I feel anxious** all of the time?

✓ **Do I have difficulty with my memory?** Do I forget where I park my car?

TABLE 2. MARKERS OF HEALTH

There are no magic numbers to look at for good health. Not all stressors will show up in the blood tests. However, here are 10 markers that we feel are good for baseline testing, which we often follow after interventions are made:

1. **Body Composition/** percentage body fat
2. **Body Mass Index** *(BMI)*
3. **Waist Circumference**
4. **Blood Pressure**
5. **Fasting Cholesterol**/lipid profile
6. **Erythrocyte Sedimentation Rate** (ESR)
7. **C-Reactive Protein** (CRP) and **Cardiac CRP** (more sensitive for the heart)
8. **Blood Sugar**
9. **Hba1c**
10. **Fasting Insulin Level** (optional)

CHAPTER 1:

A Juggling Act: Balance, Internal Stability and Homeostasis

Homeostasis: *The tendency of the body to create*
internal stability and equilibrium, despite stressors.
It is the body's need to have balance.

HOMEOSTASIS IS THE CONCEPT that our bodies strive to stay in balance without any excesses or depletion of resources, and it is the foundation for staying healthy. No over- or under-stimulation. Balance. It is what our bodies desire, and it is vital to keeping our bodies healthy, stable, calm and free of illness.

Our bodies have many adaptive mechanisms for maintaining homeostasis. In times of stress and trauma, we activate various hormones to bring our systems back into balance. Day-to-day activities trigger these adaptive devices, a task that challenges our bodies, our minds and spirit. But often, we expose ourselves to too much stimulation, excessive stresses and overuse. Our bodies then become depleted of resources and cannot maintain homeostasis. We lose our balance—and without balance, our bodies suffer and we develop illness.

Stress comes from many places. Stress comes from pressures at home and work. It comes from what we put into our bodies such as recreational drugs or medicinal ones. It comes from the food we put into bodies. It comes from lack of sleep and overstimulation. In this modern era, we have so many external stimuli. We are continually receiving information through our computers and phones. We have the internet to answer our every question. We receive information through our smartphones that notify us of every weather change, important news bulletins and every email and text from people who want to communicate with us. We are constantly moving. Our society is always "on." We go to bed with the glow of tablets at our bedsides and wake to the buzzing of text messages and social media notifications. The stimulation is immeasurable. Each of these stresses impacts our bodies. These stresses disrupt the internal homeostasis. Our bodies have to use an abundance of resources to keep the body in balance again. But with time, those resources are lost and we become sick. This overuse leads to the onset of illness *(Consider 1).*

We have many resources in our treasure chest. Those resources are our fuel and help us balance our bodies when they are being depleted by stress. Resources are in our foods such as amino acids, omega 3 fatty acids, phytonutrients and spices. Other resources come from nourishing good gut bacteria, stimulating detox and anti-inflammation pathways with sleep, sunlight, meditation and exercise and much more. *(See Figure 1, below.)*

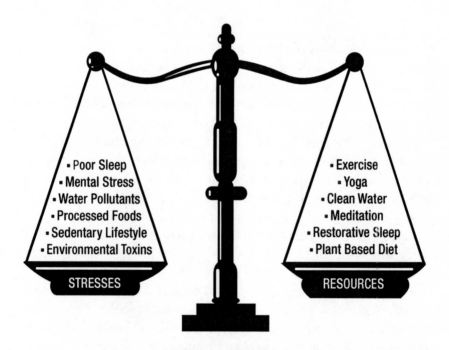

FIGURE 1. **STRESSES vs. RESOURCES**

▶ **WE STRIVE TO FIND BALANCE** between our fuel which are our resources and our toxins from our environment

Over the centuries, we have developed many new illnesses. Over time, there has been a great surge in obesity, heart disease, cancer and auto-immune disease. We are seeing more heart attacks in younger people, more lung cancers in nonsmokers and more lupus, rheumatoid arthritis and inflammatory bowel disease. One could argue that we see more of these diseases now because people are living longer and getting more age related diseases. Or one could argue that these illnesses were always there but people did not diagnose them as easily as in the past. All are possibilities. But, we have to consider as well that in the current day, there are many more toxins and stresses that our bodies are exposed to, triggering more illnesses.

Now in medicine, we have become quite advanced and have learned to treat many of these nascent illnesses. We have learned to treat cancers with chemotherapy and radiation. We have learned to treat high blood pressure with pills. We have learned to treat clogged heart arteries with pills and then stents. If the heart becomes weak, we have learned how to put in mechanical hearts and do heart transplants. If the joints go bad from excess weight, we replace the joints.

We have become a society that focuses on fixing messes instead of preventing them. We install new joints before we discuss weight loss and building muscle. We perform gastric bypass (weight loss) surgery before we educate people on what they can eat to lower their risk of obesity. We prescribe cholesterol-lowering agents and blood pressure medicines before we teach people about sodium and cholesterol, saturated fats and trans-fat. Our insurance covers anti-depressants before it covers psychotherapy. We do not focus on root causes of illness such as stress and inflammation-induced imbalances, but only the end result. With all of the advancements in health and technology, are we

> ## CONSIDER ❶
>
> ### The Stress of Always Being Connected
>
> √ **How many times do you look at your phone** when you are having a conversation with someone?
>
> √ **Do you have audio notifications** for all of your social media. Consider turning these off?
>
> √ **How often do you check your email?** How many times per hour? Can we just make a point to check them once every hour or every two hours instead of every time we hear the notification bell?
>
> √ **Consider keeping your phone away from your bed** and plan a time after which you don't look at your phone. Maybe 1-2 hours prior to bedtime will be electronics free.

any better? Are we healthier?

Now, we are at the point where we have forgotten how to prevent illness. Even as doctors, we are taught all the medications to treat illness and trained to know the surgical treatments for tumors or the arthritis-affected joints. In our current models of treating illness, there is little focus on nutrition and prevention. Most insurance companies will not pay for gym memberships, nutrition consults, or stress reduction treatments. Rather, they will pay for heart surgery, weight loss surgery and other *outcomes* of illness.

As patients we, too, look for magic pills to cure whatever ails us. We want pills that make us lose weight. We ask our doctors to prescribe pills to give us energy and make our joints hurt less. We look for pills that make our skin clear up and to treat our allergic reactions. Television commercials push medications that claim miracle cures. Even on highly rated TV shows, health professionals talk about weight loss pills and vitamins. Always, there is a pill. We have become a society that takes pills for anything and everything.

In this book, we want to focus on the root cause of illness. We want to highlight the impact of our environment on our health, and how we can change our stress responses by modifying our sleep patterns, food choices and by adding more movement to our days. We want to empower change, and provide tools that can lower our stress response whenever we think of them. We would like to give control of your health back to you.

We have developed an approach to treating ourselves that allows us to be the best we can be—free of illness, aging well with strong minds and bodies. We will give you information on how to manage bodily stress by understanding your gut health, a vital part for avoiding chronic illness, which is directly linked to the foods we choose to eat and those we avoid. We teach you to manage your external stress with mind/body techniques such as yoga, meditation and exercise. You will sleep in a world that thrives on wakefulness. You will learn how to rest and recharge.

We will not give you any magic pills, because there are no magic pills. However, we will arm you with the knowledge and tools to live long and age well. Okinawa is a group of islands south of Japan. Okinawans have long been studied for their longevity. They hold the record of having the most centenarians in the world. Not only do they achieve longevity, they also age better. They have a lower risk of chronic disease such as heart attack, stroke, cancer and Alzheimer's disease. Decades of research have linked these findings with both their diet and lifestyle. We believe with the techniques in our book, we can counteract external stressors and keep our bodies in balance. With balance, we can heal our bodies and prevent future illness. We can keep ourselves healthy and active and prevent age-related changes such as mental decline, joint pain and other age-related illnesses. With this book, we offer you tools that we use ourselves to achieve calm in a world full of activity. Let us be empowered to go on this journey together. Let us start at the beginning. *(Consider 2)* ▪

CONSIDER ❷

Broken Pill Promises

√ **Every pill** has a side effect

√ There are **no magic pills**

√ Would you rather take a **pill for every ailment** or make an intervention which has **a lasting effect?**

CHAPTER 2

How My Daughter Saved Me:

Dr. Monica Aggarwal's Story

WHEN I WAS LITTLE, I used to think that I didn't bleed. I was never injured and rarely even received a cut. When my son was born, I remember laughing at myself because of my surprise that when he fell, he would bleed. For some crazy reason, I think we all believe when we are little that we are invincible. I carried that feeling of invincibility into my 30s. I was a powerhouse. I worked hard and long hours, then came home and crashed, only to wake up and do it again the next day.

I felt I had it all. It is a tricky thing being a career woman, though. We spend our lives studying to reach the top of our game, but then that goal often coincides with the years when we want to have children. I had three children in five years. I poured the same intensity from training years into my children. I nursed them all. I made fresh meals daily, baked their birthday cupcakes and knit their Halloween costumes. I was exhausted. It was a hard life but I felt that it was a burden I had to accept in order to have it all.

After my third child was born, life changed for me. I recall the time so vividly. I went back to work eight weeks after the baby came. I remember the utter exhaustion of sleeping for three hours, going to work, then running home to nurse, cook meals and start the routine all over again. Every night, my husband would drag me out of one of our children's bedrooms so I could fall asleep in my own bed, until the next cry woke me up. I was haggard. I felt I had to sacrifice myself temporarily to have it all. One morning, four months after my third child was born, I woke up to the baby's cry and I couldn't move my right shoulder. It was red and hot. I ignored it and figured it was a trauma I couldn't remember. Three days later, my left fourth finger was red and hot. I started having trouble buttoning the kids' clothes. A day later, I felt like glass shards were piercing the bottoms of my feet.

I still ignored the pain. I started taking the elevator at work because my feet hurt too badly to climb the stairs and I couldn't bend my knees. After about a week, I knew that something was really wrong. I recall the day vividly, almost as if it was a dream. The alarm went off at 5:30 a.m. I remember feeling exhausted in my bones. I could barely get out of bed. I hobbled down the stairs to let the dog out, but my feet were worse than ever. The glass kept cutting my feet. I made it downstairs, but I could barely open the door to let the dog out. Then the baby cried. I started to run up the stairs on impulse, so as not to let the other children wake with the noise, but I couldn't get there. I couldn't run. Every bone in my body burned. I couldn't climb the stairs to reach her. I can still taste the salt in my mouth from my tears as I crawled up the stairs. I remember reaching her crib but not being able to lift her out. It was then, as I lay on the floor crying so that my husband had to pick up the baby to give her to me, that I realized I was in real trouble.

Two weeks later, I had a diagnosis of severe rheumatoid arthritis (RA). My rheumatologist looked at my inflammatory markers and told me that my prognosis would be a severe, debilitating course if I didn't begin advanced therapy immediately. After my first meeting, I was fairly sure that I would no longer be able to practice cardiology. All of the pictures from medical school of advanced RA came flooding back. The baby was now five months old and I was nursing. My rheumatologist told me to stop nursing as soon as possible because he was very concerned about the destructive signs that my lab markers portended and about how symptomatic I was. He wanted me on drugs within in one week.

So I followed his advice. I stopped nursing my baby. I cried every moment of those seven days. Every time I heard the baby cry, I had to walk away. My breasts were engorged and painful, yet I could not feed her. I still want to cry as I write this because of the deep sorrow I felt at those moments. I felt my choice was taken away from me; I had to give up something that was so dear to me. But, every patient learns quickly that you have few choices. As patients, we have to rely so much on our physicians and suspend our own disbelief.

As I started losing my hair and my daily nausea became more severe,

I felt more and more bitter and lost. I started to blame my daughter. I thought that if I hadn't had a third child, none of this would have happened. After a few months of being on the medications, though, I started to feel better. I became better adjusted to the drugs and had fewer side effects. It was around that time that I started coping with my disease, but I still hadn't released the anger. I still blamed my little girl for my disease. One day, about six months after beginning my treatment, I met a woman who would soon become a dear friend. She was a holistic nutrition consultant and was interested in educating my patients about diet. I was immediately skeptical and she offered to do my nutrition profile. It was then that I started considering the effects of the foods we eat on inflammation in our body.

It is commonly thought that people develop illness after their bodies receive multiple "insults." The first insult is often genetic, then environmental triggers add to the initial insult. For instance, a person may be genetically predisposed to heart disease (the genetic insult) and has high LDL (bad cholesterol) and low HDL (good) cholesterol levels. Then, she adds a diet rich in saturated fats and hydrogenated oils, plus a sedentary lifestyle and smoking (the environmental insults) and we have a young woman with premature heart disease. Similarly, with cancers, there is likely a genetic component, then we suffer some sort of environmental insult that creates stress (oxidative stress), which then triggers the abnormal cells to arise.

Those environmental insults/triggers can be different things to different people—lack of sleep, cigarettes, excessive sun, saturated fats, gluten, dairy. Understanding what causes their inflammation is the key. I, and others, believe that the foods we eat often trigger this inflammation. Many of us have found that simply changing the diet, cutting out inflammatory foods and adding back spices that decrease oxidative stress also lower the inflammation.

It takes time to learn our own bodies' sensitivities. Dairy and other animal products are often the source of inflammation. I was already vegetarian so I started with dairy elimination. I cried when I gave up my pizza. Like most Americans, I also worried about not getting enough calcium and protein in my diet. It took me a lot of self-teaching to understand that so much of the calcium and protein we eat comes from the beans and greens we are eating.

It has taken me four years to admit to others that I have an illness. I always felt that if I said it out loud, people would judge me or think

I was less adequate as a physician, as a mother and as a person. Now I *realize* it is because I have an illness that I understand and connect with my patients better. I can relate to their reluctance to take a medication. I feel their fear as if it were my own. I feel their helplessness and anger as the fire in my own heart. I also know now that at the end of the day, we are all affected. Then, it is about learning to avoid environmental triggers and nurturing our bodies with a plant-based diet, low in oils and refined sugars and undergoing lifestyle changes such as increasing sleep and more vigorous activity.

It has taken me a long time to embrace my disease. I have learned that it is not illness that defines us but, rather, how we respond to it that makes us who we are. A person like me who was so controlled and rigid falls hard when illness hits. I blamed my poor daughter for being the cause of my illness. I was mad for a long time. But, now I feel healthier than ever before. My cholesterol is super low. My inflammatory markers are nonexistent and I take no medications. I am strong. I just finished my first triathlon. I feel great. I have learned to take time for myself. I have learned to laugh more and not worry so much about being late or about climbing a ladder. I thank my body every day for what it has to give me and I forgive it for what it cannot. In some ways, the crazy thing is that getting sick was the best thing that happened to me. I have my girl to thank for bringing me back from a world in which I was drowning. I realize now that my daughter didn't make me sick, she saved me. ▪

CHAPTER 3

Learning the Meaning of MD:
Dr. Jyothi Rao's Story

The WHO (World Health Organization) asserts that health is not the absence of illness but it is the state of complete physical, mental and social well-being.

MY GRANDFATHER WAS A TRUE PHYSICIAN, not only because of his knowledge or clinical acumen, but because he tended to his patients where they lived and worked. He made house calls, even in the middle of the night, for treatments ranging from minor surgery to counseling—he was always ready with a warm smile or a hand to hold. He helped those in need, those without any money, those who were scared about pain and illness. In his rural community in India, he was a hero and was beloved… and I wanted to be just like him.

Visiting patients in the home is not practical but it does offer advantages. It provides the ability to see people holistically, in their life roles, and identify the stressors they encounter every day. It gives insights into their struggles about socioeconomic class, family dynamics and living conditions. My grandfather was able to identify the root cause of an ailment with much more ease since he knew, *really knew*, his patients. He made a difference in their quality of life. Ever since I can remember, I wanted to do exactly that. I wanted to help guide people to thrive. I wanted to bring some *comfort* back into their lives.

I went to medical school yearning for knowledge and eager for experience in treating illness. I pursued positions in which I would work with those who were dedicated, knowledgeable and devoted to their patients. My residency was in a tertiary care (specialized treatment) medical center where I saw a wide variety of ailments and worked alongside great and caring physicians who were leaders in their fields. I finished my residency empowered with the feeling that I now possessed the knowledge to follow in the path of my grandfather.

However, starting in private practice in New York, I was overwhelmed when I realized how little we as physicians could do to actually heal. Sure, we could diagnose illness and treat symptoms, but what about addressing the cause of the problem? Why put someone on a vigilance drug for daytime sleepiness when we should be looking for a solution to their sleep issues? We did extensive workups on many patients who had concerning symptoms, only to find everything was "normal." So, is it normal to have achiness all over? Is it normal to not have a bowel movement for five days? A city that takes pride in never sleeping provides an environment rich with stress-related symptoms such as insomnia, irritable bowel syndrome (IBS), migraines, palpitations and many more.

Why is weight gain such a big problem? Where is the joy and vitality in everyone? There was not enough time to counsel or delve deep into sources of stress, which I felt was the root of 75 to 80 percent of what I see in internal medicine. What happened to bringing *comfort* back into our patients' lives? After all of my study and hard work and aspirations to help people, all I had in my toolbox were bandages. I wrote prescriptions and briefly discussed exercise and diet. I was a fireman, putting out fires that had already started, and doing nothing to prevent future fires from igniting.

It was at this point that I decided to train in acupuncture, so that I could offer more wellness tools to my patients. I learned about the concept of energy movement and began looking at the root cause of illness. Using acupuncture in my practice gave me a new paradigm shift. It was not only a tool for common symptoms such as back pain, migraines, acid reflux and many other everyday illnesses I was treating, but I heard from patients that they felt more energetic, they slept better and their mood improved. As I learned about *creating balance,* I felt empowered once again. I could teach my patients about *elementary prevention,* which is keeping systems in balance so illness doesn't have a chance to strike. I was finally on the path to integrative, functional medicine.

No longer do we have to feel that we are destined by our genes. We have the tools to impact the ways in which our genes manifest themselves. Functional medicine allows me to delve into genetic variations, the impact of oxidative stress, nutrient imbalance and how different environmental toxins break down our bodies, according to varying socioeconomic conditions and climate exposure. These differences change the ways our bodies respond to stress and create oxidative stress and inflammatory changes. These pathways of inflammation lead to our symptoms and to different disease states.

I learned about homeostasis, or "steady state," which is the key to true healing. This is the balance of everything in our lives and our bodies. It is the balance of sleep and wakefulness, our hormones, and diets rich in high nutrient foods, unrefined carbohydrates, beneficial oils and proteins. Homeostasis also includes balance of work and home life. I appreciated the simple things such as the value of spending time in natural sunlight (with sunscreen of course)! The concept of lifestyle changes for healthier living is empowering. Anyone can use it at any time. When the body is in balance, it is more equipped to handle change and any incoming insults.

The WHO (World Health Organization) asserts that health is not just the absence of illness; it is the state of complete physical, mental and social well-being. In my opinion, this is the goal of the integrative physician: not only to diagnose and treat symptoms but to give patients their own unique and individualized tools to help them achieve an optimum state of health. It was in my post-graduate years that I learned how to keep people well. It is my goal to educate people about the multitude of various stressors in our lives, ranging from the environmental (poor air and water quality, extreme climate changes, poor food quality with pesticides, GMO and processed foods), to the chemical (toxins in water and medication side effects) to the mental (feeling out of control).

I continue to strive to find tools that allow me to practice medicine the way my grandfather did—holistically. I continue to search for knowledge that will empower my patients. Aging is an inevitable part of life. I want to teach my patients not to fear it but to embrace aging. We may not be as fast, our joints may feel creaky and we may have more wrinkles on our faces. But we can be strong. We can be at peace and free of chronic illness. It is all about balance. We will help you learn as we have been learning. The road is hard and sometimes, it is hard to see the endpoint. But, your life will be your proof. How you feel will be your motivation.

We wrote this book to provide people with tools to protect their bodies and minds so we can all live fruitful, independent lives and reduce the risk of getting chronic illness. It is about being proactive, not waiting for your systems to break down. These prescriptions are the true tools for staying well, or for bringing balance back into your body and restoring damage from inflammation and oxidative stress. This book is a guide to use along with advice from your health care provider, and to give you the tools you'll need to enjoy the life you dream of. ∎

CHAPTER 4

Breaking Down:

When balance is disrupted, stress and inflammation are created

W E NOW KNOW that imbalance in our bodies can cause illness. Now, let's understand which factors create imbalance in the first place.

Imbalance is prompted by stress and can be brought on by an injury, anxiety, toxins we ingest, lack of activity and many more triggers. The powerful effect of stress on your body is the most important concept that we will relay to you because if you recognize how stress works, you can then start the healing process.

The term "stress" was coined in the 1950s by Dr. Hans Seyle, a pioneer in the field of endocrinology. Some consider him the first researcher to examine the biological impacts of stress and the connections between the mind and body. He defined stress as a body's response to a demand for change. Stress can be emotional, mental, physical, chemical or environmental. It can be a physical reality or created in our minds, but in either case it sets off a fixed reaction in our bodies. Seyle broke down stress into "eustress" and "distress."

Eustress is good stress driven by positive anticipation, such as when we are expecting a child, or we're starting a new job or planning a vacation. It refers more to the way our body reacts to stress. It gives us good coping skills and makes our senses hyperacute. Distress, on the other hand, is negative stress and triggers inflammation and oxidative stress. Distress occurs when we suffer the loss of a child or spouse, termination of a job or divorce. Both situations demand that the body change. *(figure 1) (Consider 1)*

FIGURE 1 **TYPES OF STRESS**

EUSTRESS
Positive Stress

- Anticipation
- Expecting A Child
- Getting A Promotion
- Changing Jobs
- Planning to Travel

DISTRESS
Negative Stress

- Death
- Loss of Job
- Time Pressure
- Criticism/Bullying
- Illiness

Dr. Seyle was a pioneer because he saw the connection the mind has over the body. He formed our current thinking around the *general adaptation syndrome,* or the ways in which our bodies cope with stress. During times of changing environment or a perceived threat, our acute stress response is adaptive and allows us to cope and respond appropriately to survive the stress. An acute stress response in healthy individuals is a good thing. It is a normal process, and it is protective.[1] In the acute stress response, we see activation of the nervous system, cardiovascular, endocrine and immune systems. The goal of the stress response is to release resources for the body to make energy for immediate use. The body also starts to allocate these resources to specific organs and shut down resources to other organs to help conserve energy.

When our senses perceive a threat, the autonomic nervous system is triggered. The two major components of the autonomic nervous system are referred to as the sympathetic and the parasympathetic nervous systems. These systems are regulated by neu-

> **CONSIDER ❶**
> Do you have more distress or eustress in your life?

rotransmitters, or chemical signals, which communicate to the nervous system to set off a chain of responses. They work in balance to affect many systems of the body such as heart, eye, stomach and genitals.

The sympathetic nervous system (SNS) is also called our fight-or-flight system. The SNS triggers the release of neurotransmitters such as epinephrine and norepinephrine which then signal the cardiovascular system to increase the blood pressure and heart rate. The heart pumps faster and gets blood to all essential organs quicker so the body is ready for whatever comes its way. It also suppresses gut motility and the urge to urinate so that we aren't hungry when we are running and do not have the urge to urinate or defecate. The SNS also increases blood flow to our skeletal

Figure 2 — **Breakdown of the Autonomic Nervous System**

The parasympathetic nervous system is responsible for rest and digest.
The sympathetic nervous system is activated in times of stress
and is termed the fight or flight system.

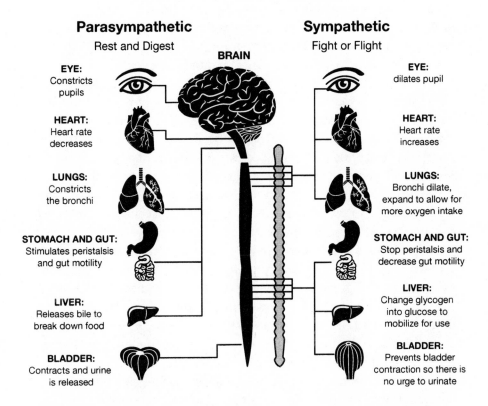

Parasympathetic
Rest and Digest

BRAIN

Sympathetic
Fight or Flight

EYE:
Constricts
pupils

EYE:
dilates pupil

HEART:
Heart rate
decreases

HEART:
Heart rate
increases

LUNGS:
Constricts
the bronchi

LUNGS:
Bronchi dilate,
expand to allow for
more oxygen intake

STOMACH AND GUT:
Stimulates peristalsis
and gut motility

STOMACH AND GUT:
Stop peristalsis and
decrease gut motility

LIVER:
Releases bile to
break down food

LIVER:
Change glycogen
into glucose to
mobilize for use

BLADDER:
Contracts and urine
is released

BLADDER:
Prevents bladder
contraction so there is
no urge to urinate

muscles and our brain. Our eyes dilate so we can see better in the dark. All of our senses become keener, we are more alert and our muscles can endure. Simultaneously, the parasympathetic (PNS), our rest and digestive system, is suppressed. This system is responsible for lowering the blood pressure, lowering the heart rate and improving gut motility. When there is an acute stressor, activities not essential for immediate survival and digestion, growth and reproduction are suspended.[2]

Another major cascade that occurs when stress is perceived is a signal in our brain to trigger the release of cortisol (from the adrenal gland, the stress response center). Cortisol has two main jobs. The first is to help make energy. It is responsible for breaking down fat (lipolysis) and making sugar from storage sources (glycogenolysis). It also mobilizes fat from the periphery to the center to prepare it for use.[3] *(figure 2)*

Its second role is to regulate the immune system. Without over-whelming ourselves here with the immunology, the role of cortisol is to balance inflammation with anti-inflammation. Our acute stress response allows for an increase in white cells—the infection fighters (macrophages and natural killer cells) that go into tissues such as our skin or other organs and act as protection against those cells most likely to suffer damage during an insult. Our immune system recruits chemicals in our blood to help fight against new trauma, infection or injury.

One of the benefits of cortisol in acute stress is that it suppresses our pain response. When we are being chased, we cannot worry about the pain in our muscles or minor injuries. This is a protective benefit. It allows us to run despite injury. Cortisol is also known to be a catabolic hormone, which means it breaks down parts of our body, such as our muscle and bone to provide nutrients to help us weather a stressful time. Again, when we are running from a tiger, we need all of the energy we can muster to save our lives. Cortisol is responsible for keeping us moving in times of stress. *(figure 3)*

People often ask whether cortisol is good or bad. Cortisol levels are a measure of stress. They are cyclic in the body. When we first wake up in the morning, our cortisol levels are at their highest. It is believed that those high amounts are needed then to mobilize our bodies for the day.[4] A way to think about cortisol is that it gives us our "get up and go" and allows us to be prepared for whatever our day holds. In a healthy state, the levels gradually decrease during the day.

However, in times of external stress, the cortisol levels shift and they become elevated at times where they would normally decline. This is necessary to activate our fight- or-flight response, to mobilize energy and allow us to meet the demands of a stressful day. Imagine a mother watching her child in a park and she witnesses him falling from the monkey bars. She sees her child on the ground, crying in pain and unable to walk. Her alarm phase kicks in and she is mobilized to get her child help. We can see then that the stress response is extremely important.

CHRONIC STRESS RESPONSE

WHEN IS STRESS DETRIMENTAL to our health? If stress becomes persistent, then our cortisol levels become chronically high. With the case of the mother who watches her child fall from the playground equipment, she learns her child has a

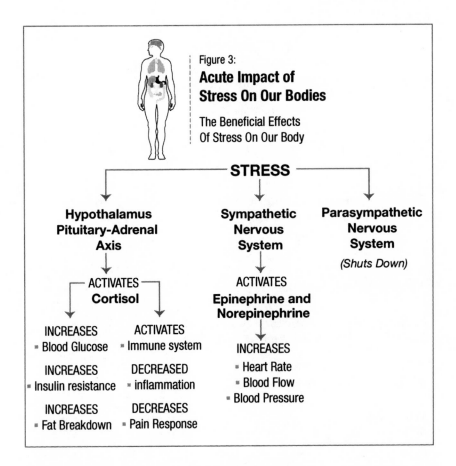

Figure 3:

Acute Impact of Stress On Our Bodies

The Beneficial Effects Of Stress On Our Body

STRESS

| Hypothalamus Pituitary-Adrenal Axis | Sympathetic Nervous System | Parasympathetic Nervous System *(Shuts Down)* |

ACTIVATES **Cortisol**

ACTIVATES **Epinephrine and Norepinephrine**

INCREASES
= Blood Glucose

ACTIVATES
= Immune system

INCREASES
= Heart Rate
= Blood Flow
= Blood Pressure

INCREASES
= Insulin resistance

DECREASED
= inflammation

INCREASES
= Fat Breakdown

DECREASES
= Pain Response

broken bone in his leg and she must fully care for him for six weeks while he is in a cast. This results in high, persistent cortisol levels with constant activation of her fight-or-flight response. Her heart rate and blood pressure are continuously elevated. Her muscles are broken down and fat is pulled from the periphery. *(figure 4)*

People with high cortisol levels often have trouble with excessive abdominal weight (apple shape). Their sugar levels are also chronically elevated. The immune system becomes over-activated and this can lead to suppression of key immune functions. This suppression can lead to increased risk for infections. Have you noticed, in times of stress, that you are more prone to getting a cold?

If the stress is ongoing, exhaustion sets in, preventing us from adjusting to the stressful situation. This is where the stress response takes the form of burnout, overtraining or exhaustion. In the case of our mother from the playground, she has poor sleep, poor support and poor nutri-

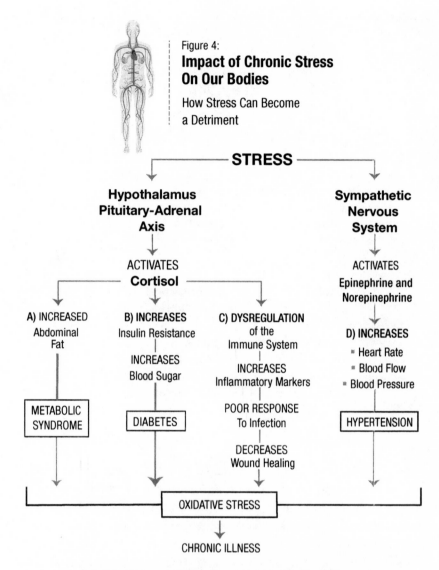

Figure 4:
Impact of Chronic Stress On Our Bodies

How Stress Can Become a Detriment

STRESS

Hypothalamus Pituitary-Adrenal Axis

ACTIVATES
Cortisol

Sympathetic Nervous System

ACTIVATES
Epinephrine and Norepinephrine

A) INCREASED Abdominal Fat

B) INCREASES Insulin Resistance

INCREASES Blood Sugar

C) DYSREGULATION of the Immune System

INCREASES Inflammatory Markers

POOR RESPONSE To Infection

DECREASES Wound Healing

D) INCREASES
* Heart Rate
* Blood Flow
* Blood Pressure

METABOLIC SYNDROME

DIABETES

HYPERTENSION

OXIDATIVE STRESS

CHRONIC ILLNESS

A, B, C, D all trigger oxidative stress which triggers chronic illness

ents which can leave her burnt out after six weeks of constantly caring for her child.

In times of burnout, there is significant imbalance in the immune response. We see more inflammatory markers, decreased wound healing and poorer response to infection.[5] Further, it has been shown that in chronic stress, there is over-activation of the hormonal systems and subsequent formation of disease-causing free radicals. Free radicals are toxic to our cells. Their formation and injury to cells is called "oxidative stress."[6] Inflammation and oxidative stress can then cause chronic fatigue, depression and excessive weight gain. In addition, persistent elevation of cortisol can lead to insulin resistance, which can cause chronic disease states such as diabetes and cardiovascular disease. Chronic stress can lead to higher levels of anxiety, increased depression and insomnia. Other functions such as cognition, memory and reproduction are also adversely affected.[7] *(Consider 2)*

Remember that cortisol is about the balance between inflammation and anti-inflammation. In chronic stress, that balance is disrupted and even with the high levels of cortisol, the body becomes resistant and the balance with anti-inflammation is lost.[8] This can cause a marked increase in inflammatory cells and can trigger an autoimmune disease in which the body actually starts attacking itself.[9]

Cortisol plays a role in aging as well. First, let's discuss how aging affects our body. Aging is defined as the process of growing old and this involves every cell in our bodies. Chronologic age is the number of years we are alive but a per-

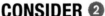

CONSIDER ❷

√ **Do you get sick** more often when you are stressed?

√ **If your memory** is worse when you are stressed

son's biologic age may be different, depending on different insults to our systems. That is why we see "age-related" illnesses at different ages in different people.

All cells in our body are continually dividing. It is a necessary function of life. All cells have genetic material in them which tell the cells their jobs. The genetic material, our genes, defines who we are and how we think. Genes are made up of chromosomes which hold that information. As cells divide, they shorten. Chromosomes have caps on the ends called telomeres whose job, over time, is to make up for the shortened chromosome length. Telomeres have a very important job, then, to make up for the loss of cell size. However, as we age, the telomeres shorten and they cannot keep up with the shrinkage of our cells and ultimately, our cells stop dividing. Without cell division, the body cannot repair and is prone to illness and dysfunction. This expedites biologic aging. Chronic stress is associated with shorter telomere length, which then causes cells to stop dividing and ultimately, is then associated with increasing biologic age and earlier onset of "age-related" illnesses[10]

Consider what age-related illnesses can do to us. With age, our lung capacity is reduced, digestive enzymes in our guts decrease, our brain size can shrink and the cushions between the disks in our spines can grow smaller, making us actually lose height. Functionally, as we age, cognitive function diminishes. Our vision weakens as well as other senses such as smell and hearing. Our fat/muscle ratio grows, causing our metabolism to slow down. Collagen in the skin dwindles and our skin thins. Our immune system becomes weakened and sleep disturbances increase. Stress can exaggerate the rate of our physical decline. In general, as we age, the risk of chronic disease grows. We desperately need tools to help lower our stress response if we want to slow aging of our cells.

Stress in our modern world comes from so many venues. When we are busy we don't have time to exercise, so we sit for most of the day. We sleep less and when we are tired during the day, we drink caffeine to keep ourselves going. We are also less accepting of others and because we spend so much time on electronic media, we are desensitized to tragedy. We walk past televisions that show war and devastation. We have less tolerance and compassion.

Always on, always multi-tasking. *(Consider 3)*

With constant stimulus, are we at our most efficient? Consider a cheetah who runs to pursue his prey. After he catches the prey, he spends time resting and recharging. That rest and recharge time is the counterbalance to the flight-or-fight response and is essential for healing the body. It is during this time that the parasympathetic nervous system is activated and the blood pressure and heart rate slow down. Our hunger response returns and digestion returns to normal. Our pain response comes back and we can spend time healing our wounds. Our cortisol levels drop as well, so we stop breaking down muscle and fat; we can again build our fat and muscle stores. We return to having a normal immune response to insults.

Now, in our current day-to-day with constant motion, work stress and overstimulation from our electronic devices and poor nutrition that causes the body aches, lack of activity and lack of sleep, our bod-

---

CONSIDER

√ **What stresses do you have in your life which are triggering your inflammation?**

* Consider where you multi task in your life.

* Do you stand and eat your dinners?

* Do you do other things while eating?

* Do you take on more work/ activities than you can handle?

ies are under constant stress. Imagine if your phone battery showed a 7-percent charge rate; you would panic. Your primary mission would be to find a charger. Think of your body that way. It needs a battery charger and if we don't have time to rest and recharge, we are prone to an inflammatory state that cannot recover from injury. We cannot heal. This is the state within which most of us lead our lives. When you read Dr. Aggarwal's personal story, you will see that she certainly was over-stressed. And with that condition came illness, as it often does. Most of us don't see how stress and overstimulation affect us until we have suffered real injury. ▫

YOUR PRESCRIPTION:

Some stressors are good and protective. **Too much stress** can be toxic and inflammatory.

Stress can be:
- Mental
- Physical
- Environmental

Learn to identify your eustress from your distress.

❶ **Think about saying 'no' to more requests** during the week to allow time to relax and recover on weekends

❷ **Schedule fewer activities** for yourself and your family to allow for more personal time

❸ **Learn to outsource** where able

❹ **While eating:** Chew slowly. Eat small meals more frequently. Don't multitask with eating

❺ **Don't check your email every five minutes.** Concentrate on checking only once per hour

❻ **Turn off computers/electronic tablets/phones** 1-2 hours before bedtime to allow the mind to calm down

See Figure 1: Eustress versus Distress (see page 30)

CHAPTER 5:

Chronic Illness is Born

*What we know about illnesses and risk factors
for illness your body can tell us*

CASE 1: Patient HB is a 39-year-old man who is a physical education teacher in a high school. *He weighed 326 pounds. When he came to see Dr. A, his blood pressure was in the 190/70 mmHg range (very high). His LDL cholesterol was 160 gm/dL and his triglycerides were 360 gm/dL. He showed signs of prediabetes. His EKG had already changed to show strain from the blood pressure. Dr. A put him on blood pressure medications and an intensive diet. She put him on an exercise plan. He lost 100 pounds. His blood pressure came into the 120 mmHg range. His LDL cholesterol dropped into the 130 gm/ dL range and his triglycerides came down into the 150 gm/dL range (normal range). He felt like he could keep up with his students and was feeling better.*

CASE 2: JS is a 45-year-old accountant who is morbidly obese *with diabetes, hypertension and atrial fibrillation (abnormal heart rhythm). He had sleep apnea (intermittently using CPAP). He was a former wrestler and wanted to get back to it. He came to see Dr. A for preoperative clearance to treat an injured toe. Dr. A put him on medication to control his heart rate and manage his blood pressure. She insisted on compliance with the patient's CPAP. She put him on a plant-based, whole-grain diet. He was the perfect patient. He lost 65 pounds, came off of some of his blood pressure medications and decreased medication for his blood sugar. His heart rates were better controlled and he felt great. Dr. A sent him for foot surgery and after the three-month healing of his toe, he started to wrestle again. He said he couldn't believe he was wrestling again. He didn't think he would ever get back to it.*

HOW WE BECOME AT RISK FOR ILLNESS

MANY OF THE ILLNESSES WE SEE in our practices are due to a disruption in balance. Persistent, uncontrolled stress causes our bodies to become depleted of the resources that we need to thrive, and creates inflammation which is the precursor to illness. These stressors often come from environmental exposures such as the nutrient-poor foods we eat, mental stress, lack of sleep and lack of movement. The stress response can lead to imbalances in the immune system, in our heart, guts and every system in our bodies. This imbalance can exacerbate and lead to cardiovascular disease, obesity, diabetes and many other unhealthy conditions. In this chapter, we are going to explore what has happened to illness over the decades.

Heart disease and stroke are the top two killers of men and women around the world.[11] In America, heart disease deaths are followed by deaths from cancer. We are seeing more lung cancer, breast cancer, pancreatic cancer and colon cancer than ever before. We also see more Alzheimer's disease, more autoimmune disease and more osteoarthritis than in years past. *(Figure 1)*

Over the decades, we have also seen our communities become more

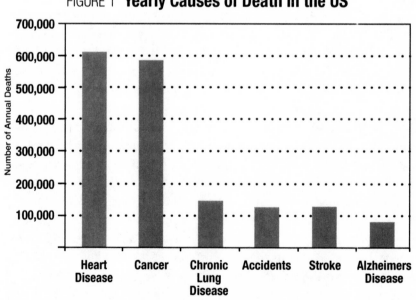

FIGURE 1 **Yearly Causes of Death in the US**

Figure 1: *Causes of death in the United States 2013*
Adapted from National Vital Statistics Report, Center for Disease Control. www.cdc.gov/nchs/data_access/Vitalstatsonline.htm

sedentary and gain more weight. Food preparation has shifted away from fresh food and cooking daily to more ordering fast food, microwaving precooked and/or pre-prepared meals. Foods are filled with preservatives to increase their shelf life. Our jobs have become more sedentary. As a society, we work more and drive home in cars instead of walking. With these changes, we are fatter than ever before in history,

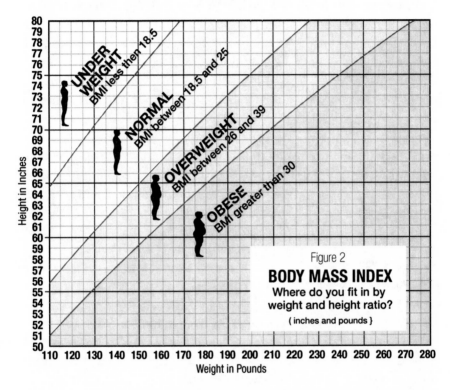

Figure 2

BODY MASS INDEX

Where do you fit in by weight and height ratio?

(inches and pounds)

with 16.9 percent of our youth and 34.9 percent of adults being obese.[12] More than two of every three adults are overweight or obese.[13] With that, the number of people with diabetes and pre-diabetes has reached 86 million, which is 36 percent of the population.[14] *(Figure 2)*

Let's talk for a moment about these illnesses in more detail.

DIABETES

DIABETES PUTS US AT SIGNIFICANT RISK FOR HEART DISEASE. We often find that people don't understand why diabetes is dangerous. When we discuss diabetes, we usually are talking about type II diabetes, which is associated with obesity and insulin resistance.

The pancreas is an organ in our bodies that makes insulin; it's needed for the glucose to be taken into cells to build fat stores for later energy use. All hormones need receptors, which are like entry cards, to get into a cell so that they are able to do their jobs. In the case of obesity or excess fat, there can be masking of the receptors on the cells and the insulin hormone is not allowed to attach to the receptor. This is called insulin resistance. The sugars become less responsive to the insulin. They don't get entry into the cell and aren't turned to fat. As a result, more sugar is floating around in the bloodstream and not going into the cells for storage. Some people might see that as positive. "If I can eat and not have it turn to fat, that's a good thing right?"

Unfortunately, no. The problem is that the floating sugars are extremely inflammatory, so as they circulate through the body they irritate your blood vessels. They cause fissures in the blood vessels of the heart and causes scabs or plaque to form. The plaque migrates to the eyes and damages their small blood vessels, so people slowly lose their vision. As the scabs build in the blood vessels, they prevent blood from flowing to the various organs. Eventually, one of those blood vessels is completely blocked and a piece of the organ that the blood vessel supplies will die.

> **CONSIDER**
>
> √ Consider what you are doing to your body to put yourself at risk for diabetes.

Studies show that weight loss can decrease blood sugars and correct diabetes.[15] It seems, then, we have the ability to change the course of the disease. Even though we may be obese, we can change our cardiovascular destiny. We can lower our risk of heart disease if we lose weight. Unfortunately, diabetes is becoming more prevalent in the United States because we are getting bigger, eating more processed foods and sugars and we are less active. *(Consider 1)*

HEART DISEASE

Let's talk about heart disease a little more, beginning with how it develops. Cardiovascular disease, often referred to as coronary artery or heart disease, is the formation of plaque in the blood vessels (pipes) that actually sit on the heart and supply the heart with blood to allow it to pump. This plaque formation, in turn, prevents blood flow through those heart pipes and subsequently prevents the heart from pumping blood to the rest of the body. Without the heart pumping, there would be no blood flow to the brain and other essential organs and we would die.

So, keeping the coronary arteries in good health is key to overall health.

The endothelium is the inner layer of cells in all blood vessels, including the pipes in the heart—the coronary arteries. The endothelium is responsible for dilating the blood vessels to accommodate changes in activity level. When we exert ourselves, our blood vessels widen to allow more blood to flow through them, so it can reach the organs that need it. When we develop risk factors for heart disease such as high cholesterol, high blood pressure or smoking, the endothelium of the blood vessels becomes damaged. This concept is termed endothelial dysfunction, which is the beginning of atherosclerosis (also known as coronary artery disease or heart disease). When the endothelium is damaged, it becomes rigid and does not dilate easily.

This damaged endothelium becomes a site for more plaque being deposited. Then the platelets (the clot makers) come to the site because they see this damage to the blood vessel, and they start repairing the lining. This process of endothelial dysfunction and subsequent platelet adhesion creates the beginning of an atheromatous plaque, or plaque forming on the insides of our artery walls. Think of this plaque like a scab on our bodies. But unlike the outer surfaces our bodies, where it does not matter how big the scab is because space is infinite, in a blood vessel it matters a great deal because the larger the scab, the more the blood flow is obstructed. Blood can't get where it needs to go. *(figure 3, page 44)*

As we develop more risk factors or the ones we have progress, more plaque adheres to the scab and it gets bigger and bigger. When the plaque closes off the blood vessel completely, a person has a heart attack. That is the more "benign" heart attack because it is a gradual process and the body has had a chance to compensate over time by slowing down. The more serious heart attack happens when one of those smaller scabs randomly ruptures (explodes) in the blood vessel and goes from a 30 percent blockage of the blood vessel to 100 percent blockage. That is the acute heart attack and often results in death or heart failure.

The late actor James Gandolfini died of such an attack. We never know which of our blood vessels is going to rupture, but we do know that inflammation plays a role. Something irritates the cap of the scab and it becomes susceptible to rupture and subsequent blockage of the blood vessel. Figuring out what causes that irritation/inflammation is key. We measure cardiac CRP (highly sensitive C-reactive protein), which is a surrogate marker of inflammation, and it tells us that the body is irritated. This is slightly different than the regular CRP (non-

FIGURE 3: **How Plaque Forms in Our Blood Vessels**

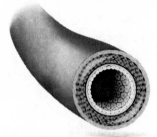

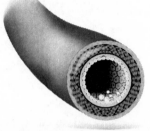

1 At birth, arteries are clear of obstructions

2 High blood pressure, smoking, high cholesterol can damage arteries walls

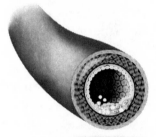

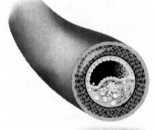

3 Scabs form, arteries grow rigid and do not dilate easily

4 Plaque builds up over time with increased exposure to poor lifestyle habits

- -

The Speed of Plaque Formation

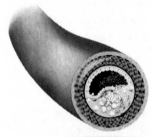

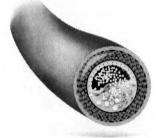

SLOW BUILD UP:
Causes chest pain and possible less severe heart attack

This is often less severe than the alternative because our bodies have had time to compensate for the decreased blood flow over time

FAST BUILD UP:
Plaque becomes irritated and ruptures, closing off the blood flow to vessel suddenly triggering *acute* heart attack

Often, these heart attacks are dangerous and most serious because the body is unprepared.

highly sensitive CRP) which is a general marker of inflammation and not as sensitive to the heart. We know that people with more inflammation are more prone to heart attacks. So our goal, as with Dr. Aggarwal's disease, is reduction of inflammation.

We know that *statins* decrease the inflammatory marker, highly sensitive CRP, and stabilize plaque. But we also think that so many things in our diet are inflammatory and cause the body to become irritated. Studies have shown that eating just one fatty meal can create endothelial dysfunction within four hours after the meal.[16] We believe that these foods are making us sick directly by causing endothelial dysfunction. The foods also cause us to gain weight and develop high cholesterol, diabetes and high blood pressure which further increase the dysfunction. We then also believe that when the foods that are inflammatory to the individual are removed, our bodies start healing. Then there are other options besides pills to make us better. More on this in chapter 7.

HIGH CHOLESTEROL

CHOLESTEROL IS AN IMPORTANT SUBSTANCE for the body. It helps build the walls of our cells. It is the foundation of our sex hormones and important for formation of myelin sheaths, which are necessary for nerve conduction. When we have too much cholesterol, however, it finds other homes, such as in our heart arteries, head arteries and legs. There are two main types of cholesterol: HDL ("healthy" cholesterol) that is responsible for removing cholesterol from the blood and taking it to the liver, and the LDL ("lethal" cholesterol) that puts it back into the blood vessel and helps to form plaque. When we are born, our LDL cholesterol is about 50 gm/dL. As our cholesterol levels go up with diet changes and other factors, we know we are more at risk for heart disease.

We often hear from my patients that their children "can afford to eat McDonald's food and fried chicken" because they are young. Is that really true? When we look at autopsies of children who died of unrelated causes, we find fatty streaks, signifying early plaque formation. Seventy-seven percent of men who fought in the Korean War had evidence of significant atherosclerosis. The average age of those men was 22 years.[17] Similar findings were seen in American men who fought in Vietnam.[18] This shows that the process starts at such a young age, and that what we put into our bodies at that young age matters. We can never afford to eat poorly. The bad foods that we eat as children put us at risk for heart disease, and as we will discuss later, for autoimmune disease, cancer and other chronic illnesses (*see chapter 6 for details*). It is so much easier to expose our children to healthy foods from the beginning and they will build a lifelong love of eating well. The habits we create in children will last for a lifetime.

OBESITY

BEFORE WE TALK ABOUT OBESITY, we need to define the terms. Obesity is often defined based on body mass index (BMI) which is weight in kilograms divided by height (in meters) squared. There are many calculators available on the internet to aid in calculating your BMI. *(figure 2).* Normal body mass indices are between 18.5-24.9 kg/m2. Being overweight is defined as body mass indices between 25 kg/m2 to 29.9 kg/m2.[19] There are gradations of obesity but for our purposes, obesity is defined as a body mass index of greater than 30 kg/m2. BMI is not a perfect assessment for obesity. BMI does not take into account thin people who have high fat percentage or heavier people who have high muscle mass. We feel fat percentage and muscle mass are more informative than BMI. However, many of the national assessments are based on BMI. As of 2009, over sixty percent of the population is considered overweight or obese.[20]

Being overweight and obese are associated with an increased risk of death.[21] In studies of overweight individuals above 50 years of age, there was nearly a 20-50 percent increased risk of dying. Mortality is proportional to amount of weight gain.

What is it that our overweight and obese population is dying of? In one study, overweight men and women had a 52-percent and 62-percent risk, respectively, of death from cancer.[22] According to the Prospective Studies Collaboration analysis,[23] when obese patients were examined, a proportionately increased risk of heart disease, diabetes, cancer and lung disease was found. Cancers associated with increased weight in particular are liver cancer, kidney cancer, breast, endometrial (uterine), prostate and colon cancer. On the other hand, there are multitudes of studies to corroborate that the leaner we are, blood pressures decrease, sugars become more controlled and we feel better.[24]

Obesity is strongly associated with high blood pressure (hypertension) and high cholesterol. Obese patients typically eat more saturated fats and highly salty foods which are felt to be significant causes of not only obesity but also of worsening blood pressure and high cholesterol. More than 100 million American adults, about 33 percent of the total adult population, have total cholesterol levels greater than 200 mg/dL (ideal is less than 200 mg/dL).[25] Of people with high cholesterol, about 67 percent of them are either overweight or obese. Seventy million American adults, 29 percent of the population, are now or have been treated for hypertension.[26] Of those people, 77 percent are either overweight or obese.

Hypertension causes damage to the blood vessels and high cholesterol boosts plaque formation. Both are directly linked to increased risk of heart disease. In the Framingham study, obese patients had more than twice the risk of heart disease compared to their leaner counterparts.[27] Obese patients are more likely to have weakening of the heart or heart failure, as well as abnormal heart rhythms.

There is also a link between obesity and stroke, liver disease and arthritis. The more weight we carry on our joints, the more traumas those joints suffer. Arthritis is one of the most costly morbidities associated with obesity. We have even linked skin changes, such as thickening of the skin (acanthosis nigricans), stretch marks and increased hair production in women, to obesity.

We weren't always so fat. We can all recall that when we were younger, people were smaller. When Dr. A was 20 years old, she weighed 120 pounds and wore a size 4. Three babies and 15 years later, She now weighs a bit more than that, but she still wears a size 4. Why is that? This is called vanity sizing. Retailers have gotten smarter. As people gained weight, they didn't fit into their usual sizes and needed bigger clothing but people didn't want to buy larger sizes, so they didn't buy as many clothes. As such, clothing manufacturers have adjusted their sizes to allow consumers to buy smaller-sized garments and feel skinnier. We heard a great article on National Public Radio (NPR) stating that a size 6 in 1970 would be comparable to a size 2 in 1996 and a size 0 in 2012. Size 0! As we have gotten larger, we have changed our conception of what is "normal." We have altered the charts of our children's growth curves to reflect the changing sizes of our youth. We are changing the sizes of our clothes to reflect that change, so we don't feel we are bigger. But we know that we are.

Many environmental factors contribute to obesity. Large portion sizes, high-sugar drinks, fast food, decreased physical activity and watching more television are all linked to obesity. Television has been shown to directly influence our risk of obesity and these trends are likely to follow into adulthood.[28]

Back in the old days, when a large number of us were farmers, we were not an overweight population. We worked in the fields all day, picked our food for supper from the garden, and ate it while it was fresh. We ate more vegetables, fruits and nuts. We lived off the land and only killed what we needed to feed our families. Nothing was wasted.

Over time, we have left our farms. We go to fast-food restaurants to get a quick meal as we drive to work. We sit for eight to ten hours per day and get up only to refill our sodas and eat meals. Often, we are so busy in meetings that food is brought into meetings. We eat what is there and often much more than we need. We eat snacks and desserts because they are readily available. We then drive home and are usually too tired to exercise. We might eat a quick frozen dinner in front of the television and fall asleep. We snack until the late hours of the night. The sizes of our plates have gotten larger so we eat more food. We drink less water and supplement with sodas and coffee to keep us awake because we are often tired. We eat pasta and simple sugars all day so we have constant dips and plateaus in our energy levels. We then go get a jolt of caffeine to keep us awake during the post-eating dips. Over time, we have become overweight and sedentary.

We have the ability to change this. Now that we have talked about the changes in chronic illness over time and the diseases our bodies are at risk for, we want to shift attention to the link between what we eat and how it changes the composition of our gut flora, which in turn activates abnormal body responses. ▪

CHAPTER 6:

The House of Bugs

Learn about your gut

CASE: A 56-year-old woman with Diabetes *was recently admitted to the hospital for persistent, foul-smelling diarrhea. Recently, she had recurrent urinary tract infections and had been prescribed multiple courses of antibiotics. She was losing weight and had low energy. She was diagnosed with C. Difficile colitis (and infectious inflammatory overgrowth in her gut) and was given more antibiotics to heal the infection of her gut. Despite multiple attempts at curing the infection, her diarrhea became intractable. She was given a fecal transplant which is when the stool of a healthy family member is placed through a scope into the gut of the ill family member. Within weeks, the patient felt better; she was eating and no longer had diarrhea.*

LEARNING ABOUT THE GUT is extremely important because you will soon learn that the bacteria in the gut are responsible for much of the immune system defense of our bodies, and also are responsible for many hormone and mood regulators. First, we need to go through some important definitions: *Microbiota* is the term that refers to all of the microorganisms (tiny bugs) in our bodies that are exposed to the outside surfaces. This includes all the bugs in the gastro-intestinal organs (mouth to anus), nose, ears and on the skin and genitals. These microorganisms are bacteria, protozoa, fungi and even viruses that inhabit our bodies. It is estimated that 90 percent of cells (approximately 100 trillion cells) found in our bodies are not human, but come from 40,000 bacterial strains. Imagine, then, that we are only 10 percent human and the remainder is bugs!

Every bacterium in our bodies has its own genetic material. The *mi-*

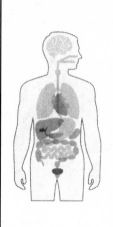

Figure 1:
What is the MICROBIOTA and MICROBIOME.

MICROBIOTA:
Microorganisms (tiny bugs) in our bodies that are exposed to the outside surfaces. These include the gastro-intestinal organs (mouth to anus), skin, nose, ears and genitals.

MICROBIOME:
Entire gene pool found in our bodies, so it includes the DNA (the brains) of every bug in our gut.

crobiome, then, is defined as the entire gene pool found in our bodies, so it includes the DNA (the brains) of every bug in our guts. *(Figure 1)* Some people call this microbiome our "second genome" or our second brain. Not only are the "human" genes outnumbered by the genetic material from our microbiota, it is likely that the microbiome has more influence on our overall health. There are many host-bacteria interactions involving signaling between multiple organ systems, including the central nervous system. The term gut-brain axis refers to the connection between our true brain and our gut brain. There are products/metabolites produced by these gut bacteria that are only available to the hosts because of the microbiota. More data is becoming available that gives us insight into the composition of the microbiota and its impact on how the body works and how it fights infection. We are learning about the role of the gut in how we act and how we think.[29]

The human microbiome project is an NIH-funded project that focuses on understanding the role of the microbiome in our bodies. This project has given us a lot of important information on the role of the gut in how we feel and how we respond to illness. From this project, we know that the microbiota plays a critical role in building and maintaining our immune system. Many people call the gut the 'internal health monitor.' It is responsible for monitoring bacteria and viruses that come into the mouth with everything we eat and preventing those infections from getting into our bloodstream and becoming systemic diseases. The gut is involved in production of vitamins, essential amino acids and fatty acids. It also impacts how our bodies utilize fats and sugars, which are important in understanding how we gain weight.[30] (Consider 1)

The presence of an intact microbiota directly impacts the health of the host. Similarly, then, having a weakened microbiota puts our bodies at risk for illness. The proliferation of the wrong kind of microbiota may predispose us to autoimmune disease, inflammatory bowel disease, obesity, infection and Type I diabetes. It also likely impacts our risk for getting allergies.[31] These microbial communities change as we age and shift, based on our diets and exposures, which can lead to an over- or under-production of certain microbes. Many of us believe that this second genome plays a crucial role in deciding how healthy, or how sick, we will be.

> **CONSIDER ❶**
>
> √ How does my gut bacteria contribute to my risk of or illness or my risk of weight gain?

THE GUT-BRAIN AXIS

WHILE HIPPOCRATES SAID that all diseases begin in the gut back in 460 BC, our understanding of its importance has been relatively recent. The gut-brain axis is a concept that was established in the 1880s and establishes the connection between our brains and our guts, which occurs via the autonomic nervous system. The autonomic nervous system is a system of nerve branches that connects the brain to the other organs. It is part of the peripheral nervous system and functions as the control center for subconscious activity such as breathing, swallowing, urinating and digestion. The autonomic nervous system is divided into enteric (gut), sympathetic (fight or flight) and parasympathetic nervous systems (rest and recharge), which all play a role in regulating gastrointestinal function. These connections are established via the vagus nerve which provides fibers from the brain all the way to the transverse colon. Stimulation of the vagus nerve causes variations in the heart rate and also changes in the gut motility. Gut motility is the activity of processing our food remnants into stool and removing all the important nutrients. Slow motility would suggest slow processing of food and can be witnessed as food contents in our stool.

As we discussed previously, when we are stressed, our sympathetic nervous system becomes activated. Our senses become more acute. We see more clearly. Our hearing is more defined. We think more clearly. *(Consider 2)* Our heart rates increase so our hearts can pump more blood to essential organs. Our blood pressure increases and blood flow improves to the brain. Simultaneously, our pain sensitivity is blunted and our bladder and gut motility slow down. When we are relaxed, our parasympathetic nervous system is activated. Our heart rates slow down and gut motility increases. This makes sense because if we are being chased, we need faster heart rates and elevated blood pressure. We need heightened senses and don't want to worry about having to urinate or being hungry. We can't worry about our pain. When we

---

CONSIDER

√ How does acute stress affect your thinking? Consider how excess stress makes you feel. Have you ever felt like a deer caught in headlights?

---

are relaxed, our heart rates and blood pressures go down and we are hungry. Our bowels and bladder work. We can focus on pain and deal with it. This is an important concept in gut motility, but also it becomes relevant when we talk about day-to-day stresses and ways to recharge.

While the link between the gut and brain has long been established, it is not entirely clear how the vagus nerve actually interacts with the microbiota. The link is likely related to neurotransmitters, hormones and short chain fatty acids that are produced by the gut. Neurotransmitters and hormones are chemical signalers or correspondents that come from the brain and travel to the gut, or vice versa. Tryptophan, for instance, is produced by the gut and is involved in sleep function and a main building block of protein. Serotonin is also largely produced in the gut and is involved in mood. Most anti-depressants are selective serotonin reuptake inhibitors. They prevent serotonin from breaking down and with

---

CONSIDER

√ How many people are on a SSRI which are antidepressants whose sole job is to increase serotonin in the body? Imagine if you healed your gut how much more serotonin you would have.

---

serotonin, our mood is stabilized. Likewise, without serotonin, we suffer from depression. *(Consider 3)* Short-chain fatty acids, fatty acids produced by the gut, have been shown to improve memory and protect the brain. Only with more recent data from the germ-free (GF) hosts, however, have we been able to further understand the nerve's true impact.

The germ-free host (shown in studies performed in mice) is a host that in concept has no microbiota. These hosts are delivered by cesarean section, fed sterile milk and live in a sterile environment. In these germ-free hosts without a microbiota, there was notably more anxiety-related behavior, decreased memory and repetitive movements. Biochemical and molecular changes were also noted, such as a change in levels of cortisol (a stress hormone) and, amazingly, differences in host gene expression. This means there are certain learning and memory genes that are altered in GF hosts compared to hosts with microbiota. Data suggests that when the normal microbiota is restored or probiotics are given to these GF hosts, many of the behavioral changes such as anxiety, sociability and other biochemical processes could be reversed.[32] This is an amazing concept. More studies and human trials are needed.

We previously mentioned that many metabolites produced by microorganisms in the gut are also neurotransmitters in the brain. Along with serotonin and tryptophan, histamine, which is involved in immune responses, is also produced by the gut. Another such neurotransmitter is dopamine which is a chemical messenger that causes dilatation of blood vessels. Tryptophan is a building block for protein synthesis. It is a precursor for serotonin. It helps us sleep. These are all important metabolites produced by the gut. Interestingly, in one study, when the germ-free hosts were recolonized, the levels of serotonin and social awareness did not change, suggesting there is an age or length of time after which gut alterations have less of an impact. Importantly, the gut flora modifications had their greatest impact on people during adolescence.[33]

> **CONSIDER**
>
> √ The younger we modify our flora, the better. Start when the kids are young.

That doesn't mean, however, that changing our gut flora will not have an impact at other times. It suggests that the most impact happens in youth. This is another argument to support teaching our children good eating habits while they are young. *(Consider 4)*

The role of the microbiota can be seen in psychiatric and neurodegenerative diseases. Autism is a neurocognitive disorder that includes a spectrum of disorders associated with decreased social skills, decreased social recognition and can be associated with repetitive movements. Genetic and environmental factors are believed to play a role in presentation in this disease. A large number of people with autism spectrum disorder have associated gastrointestinal (GI) complaints. Studies vary, but we've learned that between 9 percent and 70 percent of autistic people have some GI concerns. There is recent data to suggest a link between the autism spectrum disorders and the microbiota. Germ-free mice have been shown to lack social skills and have demonstrated increased repetitive behaviors as is often seen in autism spectrum disorders.[34] Studies have shown that probiotics can decrease gut imbalance, improve these gastrointestinal complaints and decrease immune system abnormalities. Whether the probiotics can improve behavioral issues remains to be seen in large randomized controlled trials.[35]

While there is a great deal of evidence linking the gut with the brain and nervous system, the most important role that the gut may play is immune modulation—i.e., how the body interacts with pathogens (toxins). As infants, we are exposed to many pathogens, often called antigens. Some are harmful and some benign. These antigens are needed so that the immune system can mature. They trigger the immune system to create antibodies, in small amounts, that then facilitate immune system memory. We know that germ-free animals have markedly immature immune function.[36] A link has been established showing that the microbiota are needed for early immune system development and play a role in T cell maturation (T cells are the infection fighters). The microbiota has recently been shown to help in wound healing and in controlling the inflammatory response of the gut. Stresses and antibiotic exposure at young ages do affect the gut flora production and immune development. More on this later.

BACK TO THE BASICS

THE GUT IS COMPRISED OF our stomach, small intestine, large intestine and rectum. It is made of 3,000 square feet of surface area. The more surface area that is present, the better our ability to absorb and digest. The gut is made up of an abundance of intestinal villi, which are outpouchings or protrusions in the colon, responsible for absorption. The external layer of cells of these villi is our first line of defense as they are the first to be exposed to whatever comes into the GI tract. They are the pawns on our chess boards and the infantry men in our cavalry.

These cells are followed by the intestinal dendritic cells, which resemble tiny trees branching out and are often considered the first responders. These cells are the soldiers on horses. They are more equipped to handle the entry of a pathogen. Beyond that, we see the immune

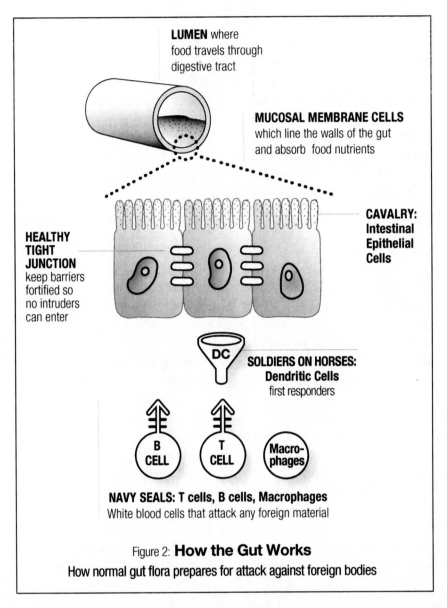

LUMEN where food travels through digestive tract

MUCOSAL MEMBRANE CELLS which line the walls of the gut and absorb food nutrients

CAVALRY: Intestinal Epithelial Cells

HEALTHY TIGHT JUNCTION keep barriers fortified so no intruders can enter

DC

SOLDIERS ON HORSES: Dendritic Cells first responders

B CELL

T CELL

Macro-phages

NAVY SEALS: T cells, B cells, Macrophages
White blood cells that attack any foreign material

Figure 2: **How the Gut Works**
How normal gut flora prepares for attack against foreign bodies

cells (the T and B cells) which are active immune fighters. These cells are the snipers and our "Navy Seals." They are the best of the best, ready to attack any foreign material that invades our bodies. As Harvard professor and pediatric gastroenterologist Dr. Alessio Fasano says, "the intestinal mucosa [gut] is the battlefield on which friends and foes need to be recognized and properly managed to find the ideal balance between tolerance and immune response." *(Figure 2)*

HOW THE GUT IS CREATED?

WHEN WE ARE BORN, we go through our mothers' vaginal canals (our birth canal) and are exposed to our mothers' microbiomes. We suck on our parents' skin. We then are nursed by our mothers and with that, are exposed to our mothers' skin flora and receive bacteria, antibodies and nutrients that her milk possesses. Soon after birth, the newborn's gut is rapidly populated with bacteria that contribute to the creation and maintenance of the epithelial barrier, aid in gut hemostasis and enhance the formation of blood vessels.[37]

We then crawl on the floor and suck on our toys. We are exposed to other people, our pets and our plants, all of which are covered in bacteria and nourish our gut. We go outside and are exposed to dirt with all of its valuable microbes. We eat the grass and lick things that our pets have licked and we obtain more bugs. This is good. Exposure to small numbers of pathogens will strengthen our immune system. Over time, however, our behaviors have changed, as explained by the "hygiene hypothesis." As we have learned the importance of sanitation and its role in infection, we clean and sterilize most everything. We know that sanitation prevents the spread of germs and because of this knowledge, we have reduced the number of illnesses that have affected our children. With greater access to medical care, we take our children into doctors with many common ailments. Antibiotics are commonly prescribed by physicians.

But have we gone too far? Is it possible to be overly clean? What is the impact of our hand sanitizers and antibacterial soaps? What is the impact on our bodies of treating all of our illnesses with antibiotics? Are we over-treating illnesses, and could many of them be just watched while our bodies work them out? We know many physicians who feel infections are viral where antibiotics don't work, but still, maybe because of pressure from patients, will prescribe antibiotics. Are we doing the right thing? With all of these changes in the modern era, we have also noted the onset of so much more allergy, autoimmune disease and inflammatory bowel disease.[38] The larger families of ages past who lived in less sanitary conditions were not afflicted with these same illnesses. What are we doing wrong?[39]

THE PROPORTIONS OF BACTERIA IN OUR GUT

BESIDES ANTIBIOTICS AND SANITIZERS, we also have proof that the foods we eat change our gut flora. In other words, certain foods foster certain gut bugs. Are some bugs better than others? A study was done in

2010 on children in rural Africa versus European children. The rural African children eat a diet that is primarily vegetarian (low in fat and animal protein), mostly comprised of lentils, millet, sorghum, black eyed peas, vegetables and spices. This diet is full of fiber and resistant starches *(Figure 3)*. Also, of note, the rural African children were typically breast fed for up to two years along with eating this diet. These rural African children have gut bacteria comprised of a high level of Bacteriodes and a low number of Firmicutes bacteria, which we explain below.

These proportions are important for many reasons. They create a bacterial balance that is associated with good weight management (more on this later). More importantly, these rural African children with the primarily vegetarian diet have more short chain fatty acids (SCFA) compared to their European counterparts. SCFAs are the byproducts of the certain bacteria in our guts that ferment fibers and resistant starches that come from our whole grains and plants and are essential to good immune function.

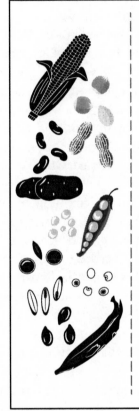

Figure 3:
RESISTANT STARCHES.

Resistant starches are complex carbohydrates that are digestible, unlike fiber, which is largely undigestible.

These resistant starches pass through the small intestine and get to the large intestine primarily in their original form. **They ferment in the colon and allow for growth of the good bacteria**.

These starches can be found in **rice, beans, seeds, corn,** as well as **potatoes, plantains** and **legumes.**

THE ROLE OF SHORT CHAIN FATTY ACIDS

THERE ARE THREE MAIN BACTERIAL TYPES that live in our gut. There are the Bacteroides, Firmicutes and Actinobacteria. When these bacteria break down plant-based foods and whole grains, they release short chain fatty acids (SCFA). It seems the ideal balance of gut bugs is to have high levels of Bacteroides and low Firmicutes, as seen in rural Africa. These bacteria appear to be very effective at processing these plant-based foods and starches to yield a good balance of SCFAs.

The main SCFAs that are produced are acetate/acetic acid (60 percent), propionate/propionic acid (25 percent) and butyrate or butyric acid (15 percent). Both Bacteroides and Firmicutes produce beneficial short chain fatty acids but it is the ratio of those fatty acids that appears to matter.[40] These SCFAs have an important role in that they provide energy to the intestinal cells and are responsible for water and electrolyte absorption. They are also important modulators of the immune system. The rural African children had a larger number of acetic acid and butyric SCFAs than their European counterparts who have more Propionic SCFAs. However, more importantly, the rural African children had decreased representation of pathogen bacteria (bad bugs such as Shigella and E. coli),[41] which means they had fewer of the bad bugs in their system compared to their European counterparts.

This study is important because it shows that what we eat impacts the bugs in our guts. Plant-based, whole grains such as those eaten by the rural African children are full of these resistant starches and build up SCFAs that help strengthen the immune system and likely put us at less risk for infectious illness. Experts are trying to isolate the exact ratios of these bacteria to determine their beneficial effects based on these studies; however, more data is needed to make firm recommendations.

The link between obesity and insulin resistance also appears to be connected to the bacteria in our colon. Interestingly, obese people have a different gut bacterial makeup than lean individuals. Obese individuals have a ratio of Firmicutes/Bacteroides that is similar to the European children. This may imply that the reversed ratio may put the European children at risk for obesity.[42] This bacterial ratio of high Firmicutes and low Bacteroides corresponds to a state of bacterial overgrowth state=bad or dysbiosis. In a study of calorie-restricted mice, the reciprocal is true (i.e. they have more Bacteroides and fewer Firmicutes). These Firmicutes are more efficient at extracting energy from food, which allows for better utilization of energy. If that energy is not utilized, though, it is quickly turned into fat. Then having fewer Firmicutes means that we need to process more food to obtain energy (i.e. more food is broken down). We know that people who eat a calorie-restricted diet have lower levels of Firmicutes and more of the Bacteroides species, which appears to be the ideal proportion. Similarly, in patients who undergo gastric bypass surgery, similar changes are found.[43] With this concept in mind, researchers have tested probiotics to manipulate the gut flora towards this proportion. Data shows that probiotics, often found in yogurt and fermented products, can alter the microbiome and decrease the obesity potential in animal models.[44]

Notably, we also see the same imbalance of bacteria in patients with IBD, diabetes and colon cancer.[45,46] In ulcerative colitis, for instance, there is a decrease overall in SCFAs in the host gut.[47] Butyrate or butyric acid, in particular, has been extensively studied and appears to be the main byproduct in ensuring colonic health. It has been associated with rapidly reproducing cells and immune response fluctuations. Recall that butyric acid was a significant SCFA in the rural African children compared to their European counterparts. Butyrate also appears to play a role in the release of the hormone leptin (a satiety hormone, which we will discuss at the end of the SCFA section).[48] Bottom line: A good combination of resistant starches can foster generation of the right bacteria and the optimal proportion of beneficial short chain fatty acids.

The wrong proportion of SCFAs can directly trigger inflammatory responses, specifically activating our macrophage cells. Macrophage cells are types of white cells (infection fighters) that eat up debris and bad microorganisms. Macrophages trigger inflammation and are notably increased in disease states such as diabetes, atherosclerosis, rheumatoid arthritis and neurodegenerative diseases.[49, 50]

These macrophages become activated by a stress and produce immune response hormones (TNF-, IL-1 and IL-6, chemokines, nitric oxide {NO} and arachidonic acid derivatives such as thromboxane A_2, prostaglandins E_2 and F_1). These markers are directly involved in immune response and inflammation.[51] The excess adipose tissue in our bodies is also associated with increased production of inflammatory markers (TNF-alpha). These inflammatory markers are known to mediate insulin resistance and promote diabetes in obese patients.[52] This gut imbalance, or dysbiosis, via the irregular proportions of SCFAs can then induce a state of chronic inflammation.[53] *(Consider 5)*

> ## CONSIDER
>
> √ How we eat can dictate how much inflammation we produce which is the basis for chronic illness

OTHER BYPRODUCTS OF POOR DIET

WE HAVE LOOKED AT HOW RESISTANT starches and plants affect the ratio of different types of bacteria in the gut and their role in the formation of SCFAs. Let us look a little at the converse: what does a high-fat diet do to the gut flora? A high-fat diet is associated with high levels of lipopolysacchride (LPS), another byproduct of bacterial processing. The gut bacteria make LPS in response to a high-fat diet, which then triggers a leaky gut (more on the leaky gut later).[54] Harmful infectious bacteria also can carry high amounts of LPS. Antibiotics that decrease the bacterial overgrowth also decrease levels of LPS. Similarly, certain prebiotics (foods for gut flora) and probiotics also decrease LPS. In a study of 7,000 patients with diabetes, the levels of LPS were higher than in nondiabetic patients.[55] When mice on a high-fat diet were then given probiotics, the levels of insulin resistance decreased as did the levels of LPS.[56] We know that proportion of SCFAs similar to the rural African children can suppress lipopolysaccharide (LPS) and cytokine triggered pro-inflammatory markers.[x] Importantly, high levels of LPS have also been noted in Alzheimer's disease and autism compared to healthy controls.[57,58]

LEPTIN:

WE TALKED ABOUT LEPTIN EARLIER with its relation to butyrate or butyric acid which appears to regulate leptin. Remember that butryic acid is a SCFA that has many protective effects.

Leptin is a hormone produced by fat cells (white adipose). Leptin communicates with the brain and appears to play a role in energy expenditure and food intake regulation, as well as in insulin, glucose and lipid metabolism.[59] Its job is to tell the brain that the body is satiated and has enough nutrients within it to conduct all the basic functions of living. It is often called the "satiety hormone." Leptin also has a role in reproduction and ovulation, and in immune function.[60]

It is an interesting hormone. Leptin levels are low in times of anorexia. Appetite is activated and energy expenditure goes down. This makes sense because anorexia is an energy deficient state and appetite would be heightened to increase caloric intake with the goal of increasing body mass. In animal models when there is leptin deficiency, subjects become overly hungry and gain weight. Levels then start increasing and satiety occurs. Weight is then maintained.[61] On the other hand, if an animal subject is given leptin, it will need less food, and will burn more energy and lose weight.[62]

The interesting phenomenon occurs in times of obesity. We know that with more fat cells, there is more leptin. But if the leptin levels are high, one would expect that the person would eat little and lose weight.

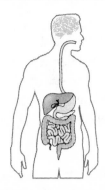

Figure 4:
LEPTIN

The role of the
hormone, **leptin**,
in our feeling of satiety

ANOREXIA, low calorie intake—activates leptin, to increase appetite and decrease energy expenditure to slow down break down of food. When we don't eat, our bodies conserve everywhere and minimize any energy expenditure.

FULL MEAL—suppresses leptin— decreases appetite and increases energy expenditure so food can be broken down.

OBESITY— large amounts of the hormone leptin is present but our bodies are not sensitive to it — leptin resistance. So despite being adequately nourished, with leptin resistance, we don't feel full.

LEPTIN RESISTANCE is triggered by obesity, overeating of simple sugars.

This, however, is not the case. If an obese person is given leptin, she does not lose weight.[63] The concept of leptin resistance is born. Leptin resistance is the idea that leptin is circulating in the body but the brain can't see it or hear its signal and doesn't know to create the feeling of satiety. People who have leptin resistance continue to eat, crave sweets and gain weight. Leptin resistance seems to run hand in hand with insulin resistance, which is a precursor for diabetes.

Recall that diabetes is a state where sugar is not easily turned into fat and instead the sugars are floating around the blood. Because the fat stores are not full in diabetes, leptin production increases. It is a double hit when you are obese *and* have diabetes because you produce high levels of leptin but your brain can't appreciate it. And when you have lots of sugar in your body that is not being converted to fat, the leptin will be activated further so your levels are higher than ever. The brain doesn't trigger satiety and the cycle continues. *(Figure 4)*

Leptin resistance appears to be due to overexposure to leptin. High levels of leptin likely blunt the brain's ability to sense it. It is believed that sweets and foods high in fructose (simple sugars) cause surges in leptin and are the mainstay of leptin resistance.[64] Then it seems that eliminating these sugars from our diet can decrease our leptin and improve our leptin sensitivity— a key to weight loss. Studies have been ongoing on leptin and its benefits. Leptin supplements have no weight loss benefit; therefore, we discourage their use.

> **CONSIDER ❻**
>
> √ Simple sugars can trigger leptin resistance. Fruit do have simple sugars. We often recommend the removal of fruits for 3 days to jump start the process. However, fruits do have many benefits like vitamins, mineral, and antioxidants and fiber so they should not be excluded for long term.

One other important point about leptin: severe caloric restriction in a diet activates leptin. The body activates leptin and creates significant hunger. Therefore, weight loss is hard to achieve with marked caloric restriction because you feel so hungry. Also, in these times, we hold onto every ounce of energy longer. Our bodies create fatigue so there is less calorie burn for self-preservation. The key to weight loss is not starving the body. It doesn't work. We feel constant hunger and excessive fatigue too. We then, should focus on eating the right foods that don't trigger leptin resistance; i.e. simple sugars. Let me say that again. If we eliminate the simple sugars in our diet then we can decrease leptin resistance.

Now, people often ask about fruits. Fruits do have simple sugars and often we recommend a short (three days) removal of fruits to jumpstart the process. However, fruits in the long term have so many benefits including vitamins, antioxidants and fiber, so they should not be eliminated for the long term. (*Consider 6*).

It is important, though, to not eat so little that you are activating leptin. Recall that activating leptin will just increase your appetite, but you will extract less energy from food. That means your body won't metabolize the food so quickly because it is trying to conserve it. Don't try to put yourself on a severe caloric restriction (unless you're under a doctor's supervision). Severe caloric restriction will make you miserable and it just doesn't work. We will teach you to lose weight and keep it off without starving yourself.

THE BYPRODUCT TMAO AND PLAQUE FORMATION

THERE APPEAR TO BE OTHER LINKS between high-fat diets, changes in the gut and effects on the overall health of the body. Studies in mice and in humans have shown a direct link between the intestinal microbiome and atherogenesis (plaque formation) in patients with diets rich in phosphatidyl choline. The main sources of phosphatidyl choline are eggs, liver, beef and pork. When these types of food are ingested, they are processed in the gut and the metabolites trimethylamine and trimethylamine-N-oxide (TMAO) are formed. In recent studies, a clear link has been identified between a diet rich in animal products and an increase in this metabolite, TMAO. Further, a link has also been established between elevated levels of TMAO and increased risk of atheromatous plaque, therefore an increased risk of major adverse cardiovascular events. This risk of triggering more such events was seen in patients with known cardiovascular disease and those without disease.[65] This is amazing because it shows an example where the foods we eat directly create metabolites that promote plaque formation.

There is a lot of speculation and thought, then, about how to fix the gut flora and suppress the production of TMAO. It is likely that probiotics and antibiotics will decrease the TMAO and will be the source of ongoing study. However, most importantly, we can just eliminate the products that increase the TMAO. A vegetarian and/or high-fiber diet has been shown to lower the amount of choline in animal subjects and therefore, reduces the amount of TMAO. (*Consider 7*)

Not only can the food we eat impact the type of bacteria in our guts, but certain food triggers can weaken the gut walls. This is called intestinal permeability, or "leaky gut." We know that chronic stresses and food triggers increase intestinal permeability and cause the intestinal villi to break down.[66] The junctions between each of the villi, outpouchings, are called tight junctions, which become loose and allow the bloodstream to be exposed to abnormal bacteria or bacterial byproducts. Those abnormal byproducts can then enter into the bloodstream and create an inflammatory response. This inflammatory response triggers formation of immune

> ## CONSIDER ❼
> √ Choline is important in nerve conduction and brain function. There are many sources of choline that do NOT come from meat products such as nuts, beans, peas, spinach, wheat germ and fish.

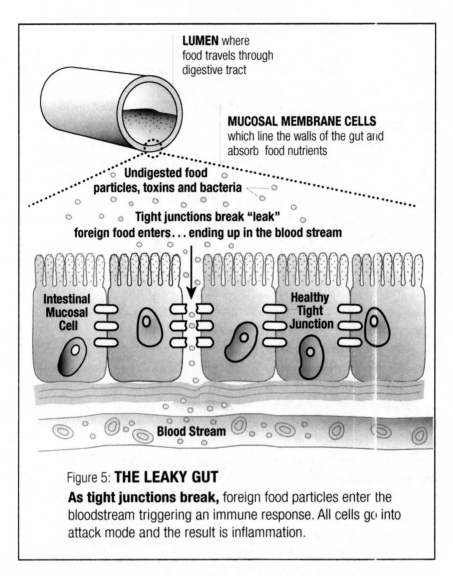

LUMEN where food travels through digestive tract

MUCOSAL MEMBRANE CELLS which line the walls of the gut and absorb food nutrients

Undigested food particles, toxins and bacteria

Tight junctions break "leak" foreign food enters... ending up in the blood stream

Intestinal Mucosal Cell

Healthy Tight Junction

Blood Stream

Figure 5: **THE LEAKY GUT**
As tight junctions break, foreign food particles enter the bloodstream triggering an immune response. All cells go into attack mode and the result is inflammation.

complexes that can attack different parts of the body.

An example of the leaky gut phenomenon is found in Celiac disease, the study of which has been pioneered by Dr. Alessio Fasano at the Massachusetts General Hospital for Children in Boston, Massachusetts. People with Celiac disease are sensitive to gluten, which is present in wheat, rye and barley. When patients with gluten sensitivity eat gluten, their bodies respond poorly. Over time, they develop symptoms of malabsorption because their guts are unable to absorb any useful food particles—the gut is too massively inflamed. They develop diarrhea, abdominal pain, failure to thrive and can have neurologic manifestations.

Dr. Fasano and others have shown that when patients with gluten sensitivity are exposed to gluten, the tight junctions between their intestinal cells become leaky. The doors to the insides of our bodies open. An environmental trigger, such as wheat in the case of Celiac disease, then comes through the door and creates an immune reaction. Immune complexes form which then destroy the villi. These villi then cannot contribute to digestion and cannot help shunt essential nutrients into the bloodstream. These immune complexes create systemic reactions. Fasano believes that some level of leaky gut is a good thing. Most people have an intestinal permeability where the doors open for a short time. During that time, the immune system gets training. But in Celiac patients, the intestine is leaky for hours and the immune system becomes massively inflamed. As Fasano says, "FRIEND OR FOE: when there is a fight, there is always collateral damage, i.e., inflammation." *(Figure 5)*

Some environmental triggers can make one person have a leaky gut for hours while another person has a leaky gut for just minutes. This leads to our understanding that a person must have a genetic predisposition to a disease. We can't necessarily fix predisposition because that is what we get from our parents. But it is only when the environmental trigger appears, however, that a person actually becomes sick. Then we can eliminate the trigger, decrease the leaky gut and decrease inflammation and treat the chronic disease. *(Consider 8)*

> **CONSIDER ⑧**
>
> √ Environmental triggers can cause a leaky gut. Most of the time that trigger is the food we eat. That food trigger is different for different people. When you eliminate the trigger, you can eliminate the inflammation.

THE LEAKY GUT

FASANO AND OTHERS BELIEVE that many autoimmune diseases are affected by food sensitivities and changes in the microbiome at an early age. The leaky gut has been associated with other autoimmune diseases such as type I diabetes.[67] Type I diabetes is one such autoimmune disease in which a patient's own immune system attacks the insulin- producing beta cells. Without insulin, our bodies are unable to process sugars and convert them to storage in the form of fat. The link between how the leaky gut triggers immune reactions that attack the pancreas in some people and cause type I diabetes, and in others creates lupus, rheumatoid arthritis or multiple sclerosis, is not clear. Each person has different genetic predispositions and environmental triggers. Importantly, there are other environmental triggers for inflammation beside diet and gut permeability; we can't ignore the roles of stress and trauma, obesity and smoking as important causes of total body inflammation.[68]

What is unclear, however, is how much of a role the imbalance in the gut bacteria has on triggering the leaky gut versus a genetic predisposition to some food sensitivity. In other words, will a food sensitivity alone trigger inflammation and illness in a genetically predisposed person or do you also need dysbiosis? We believe that you need the whole package: genetic predisposition, exposure to a sensitized food and abnormal gut flora. Presumably our gut flora changes based on what we eat, and certain gut changes make it more at risk for a leaky gut. The gut alterations and resulting high levels of LPS also seem to be associated with increased intestinal permeability, and the host immune system eventually reaches a constant state of chronic inflammation.[69] In one study, mice fed a high-fat diet exhibited higher permeability to small molecules, and reduced or altered expression of the tight junctional proteins occludin and zonulin-1.

> ## CONSIDER 9
>
> The positive impact of adding plant based diet to shifting our bugs to create more SCFA and a stronger immune system

This means that mice with a high-fat diet could not create tight adhesions between their cells; therefore they allowed bacterial byproducts to enter the bloodstream.[70] In chronic kidney disease patients we see the same sort of significant bacterial overgrowth, changes in the gut flora and evidence of disruption of the intestinal barrier.[71] We believe this is what happened to Dr. A. She had a genetic predisposition to disease. She had food sensitivity to dairy and abnormal gut flora: the perfect storm.

This information is groundbreaking and provides the first links between the changes in the microbiota and its link to intestinal permeability. The gut likely holds the key to not only treating the obesity problem, but also treating the inflammation that triggers so many obesity related illnesses. Studies are ongoing to link high-fiber diets to increased SCFAs, and determine whether that diet will reduce inflammatory conditions.[xxxvii]

We have now seen our gut flora plays a very important role in how we feel. We also know that exposures from childhood are important for keeping our bugs strong and ready to attack. We have learned that in modern times we have changed the bugs in our guts because of antibiotics and perhaps highly improved sanitary conditions. We have shown that the foods we eat can modify our gut flora, and byproducts of the poor foods have been linked to heart disease, Alzheimer's disease and autism. We also know that a whole-grain, plant-based diet helps our gut bugs to shift so that we produce more SCFAs, which are pivotal in maintaining a strong immune system and better overall health. WOW. *(Consider 9)*

This is an area of great excitement and ongoing investigation. We can take this link one step further: if we alter our diets to make them more plant-based and full of resistant starches, we will have gut flora similar to that of rural African children. We will harbor fewer dangerous bugs. We will produce more SCFAs to modulate our immune responses. And perhaps, we will lower our risks for the leaky gut. With all of these changes, we can reduce inflammation and potentially cure our diseases. A recent study shows this. It was a two-week study comparing the diets of rural African adults—diets full of fiber, starch, legumes and vegetables—with the African American (AA) diet, which was primarily fat-based. It was quite notable that the African participants' guts contained more of the carbohydrate-fermenting bacteria and higher proportions of butyrate than the AA population's guts. The African colons had significantly fewer polyps than their AA counterparts. When the diets were switched, the inflammation in the colons of the AA population significantly improved and the African population's colons grew remarkably worse.[72]

Another concept that needs to be hashed out is infection. Scientists have discovered viruses that are suppressed by different bacteria in the microbiome and others that are activated. Germ-free mice were found to be more susceptible to the influenza virus than mice with normal gut flora.[73] Similarly rotavirus, which causes a significant diarrheal illness, can be suppressed with probiotics.[74] Other viruses, however, seem to replicate within a healthy microbiome. The link between viruses and the microbiome is not completely clear and needs more work. The microbiota appears to have links throughout the body. Certain bacteria in our guts have been found to regulate the lung immune system and our ability to develop respiratory infections.[75]

One infection known as Clostridum Difficile colitis (C. diff) is an overgrowth of a type of bacteria in our guts that occurs when our native gut flora is wiped out by antibiotics. Studies show that infusing donor feces into the gut of an individual with C. diff is more effective at treating the overgrowth than any antibiotic.[76] This is some of the greatest new data showing that infusing someone else's healthy microbiota can influence the course of a bacterial illness. It's a mind-boggling discovery because it shows that giving another person's bugs to someone with a sick gut can cure a disease.

The data on the microbiome is ever-expanding. We have the framework linking chronic illnesses and the microbiome, and as more of these studies are done, the treatments of chronic illness also will change.

We may not be able to control our genetic predispositions, but we can control our environmental triggers. We can control what we eat. Common food sensitivities believed to be triggers for leaky gut are animal products, specifically red meat, dairy products, processed foods and gluten. All of these will be discussed later in this book. Often, treatment of many autoimmune diseases has to start through process of elimination and discovering each person's environmental triggers. This concept is the foundation for diet modifications that we recommend.

Many health professionals, we included, argue also that we should let natural things be natural. Do not stop your kids from eating dirt, as long as it hasn't been sprayed with pesticides. Let them get dirty. Let your dog lick the kids' faces. Don't spray everything with bactericidal soap. Don't wash your hands with bactericidal soap or use alcohol-based hand sanitizers. Unless we work in a hospital or are constantly exposed to infections, the bacteria that we are exposed to are good for our microbiota. Our intestines become strong and hardy and the intestinal barriers become strong. Nourish your bugs. Don't be afraid of them.

PROBIOTICS

PROBIOTICS HAVE BEEN DEFINED as "live organisms that when given in adequate amounts confer health benefits."[77] Probiotics have received a great deal of attention lately. It started with the concept of lactose intolerance, which is the inability of the body to break down lactose, a key component of cow's milk. As we age, the amount of lactase enzyme we produce in order to break down lactose decreases. As a result, with lactose malabsorption, people experience bloating, gas and watery diarrhea. It has been discovered that giving those same people yogurt can reduce their intolerance.[78]

Gastroenterologists and scientists have started looking at what it is about yogurt that allows people to tolerate it better than milk. In yogurt production, milk is fermented, which causes the production of lactase. Several main bacteria are produced in yogurt cultures, two beneficial bacterial strains in particular: Lactobacillus bulgaricus and Streptococcus salivarius subsp. Thermophilus.[79] Multiple studies have shown that ingestion of variable quantities of yogurt decreases lactose malabsorption and improves tolerability. In acute diarrheal illnesses, other strains of Lactobacillus have been used for treatment.

In one large, important paper, 287 children under three years of age were given a probiotic with oral rehydration therapy versus the rehydration therapy alone. Those who received the probiotic had shorter, less severe illnesses.[80] Also, importantly, in multiple studies, people who took probiotics while traveling were protected from the "traveler's diarrhea" by almost 50 percent.[81] Different strains of good bacteria were used in the various studies and a number of them were found to have benefits.

The most interesting work on probiotics extends beyond use in gut-related illnesses. In one study of pregnant women, the subjects were given probiotics prior to delivery and continued while breastfeeding or, if formula-fed, the probiotic was supplemented into the diet of the newborn. The children who had received the probiotic showed a 50-percent reduction in their eczema, and that improvement lasted for up to four years post-delivery.[82] There is also data available on decreases in dental caries (cavities) when subjects were given probiotics. Probiotics likely also play a role in inflammatory bowel disease.[83] And many animal studies and small human studies show a role of probiotics in lessening symptoms in rheumatoid arthritis patients[84],[85] and a role for probiotics in treatment of malignancy.

Trials on probiotics are few and small, however, making it challenging for physicians to recommend them on a wide-scale basis. We think the importance of probiotics is as a proof of concept. It provides us another compelling view that highlights the role of healing the gut to heal the body. We have enough data to suggest that providing the body with needed gut bacteria can decrease our overactive immune markers in rheumatoid arthritis, eczema and possibly inflammatory bowel disease and diabetes. It may play a role in cancer abatement as well. We can find few negatives to probiotics, so overall, we don't discourage them— but as you will see in the section on diet, we want you to consider natural probiotics as part of your dietary regimen. We do caution about the benefits of cow's milk-derived yogurt as the source of probiotics, as will be discussed in the next chapter.

SUMMARY:

MICROBIOME: A CONNECTION TO THE OTHER SYSTEMS in our body. It has a role in how we feel, how hungry we are and how we respond to illness.

Our exposures affect the strength of our guts. We should not be afraid to get a little dirty because it nourishes our gut bugs.

Our diet is a trigger for many changes in the gut. If we eat excess fat, we build lipopolysaccharides and create gut imbalance. We build TMAO which triggers plaque in the heart. If we eat too much sugar, we trigger leptin resistance.

If we nurture our gut bugs, we will build SCFAs which are important for our immune system and decreasing inflammation.

Natural probiotics have a role in nurturing the gut. ▪

YOUR PRESCRIPTION:
Start Being Kind to Your Gut

❶ **Don't be afraid to get a little dirty.** Avoid hand sanitizers and use plain old soap.

❷ **Avoid high fat food and meat**, which trigger bad metabolites in our bodies and produce heart plaque.

❸ **Avoid food triggers that create a leaky gut.** These are different foods for different people but can trigger chronic illness. Be aware of what food does to your body. Eliminate one at a time and listen to your body.

❹ **Avoid simple sugars** which trigger leptin resistance.

❺ **A strong gut makes a strong body.** Move towards a whole-grain, plant-based diet.

CHAPTER 7:

Heal Thy Gut:

The role of elimination

CASE 1: Jane S is a 62-year-old female who arrived at the office with shortness of breath with exertion. *She was moderately overweight with high blood pressure, very high cholesterol and prediabetes. She wasn't active and when she started a walking program, she was surprised that she was so short of breath. Dr. A noted her blood pressure was borderline high. Her EKG was normal so Dr. A did a stress test, which was normal. She suggested a diet change and a cholesterol medication. She had heard about the memory and liver issues connected with statin medications and wanted to try changing her diet before she resorted to taking pills.*

We talked about which foods she needed to eliminate. She gradually stopped eating animal fat, including dairy, over a three-month period. Her cholesterol levels came down 80 points. Her blood pressure normalized and Dr. A started taking her off of medicine. The patient lost ten pounds. She looked fabulous and hasn't looked back.

CASE 2: Robert E is a 65-year-old man *whom Dr. A has known for years. He started having rectal bleeding (bleeding out of his bottom). He became markedly anemic (low blood count) and because of the significant anemia, he started developing exertional chest pain. Even walking to the bathroom, he would feel chest pain. He was admitted to a hospital where he required 4 units of blood. The doctors did an endoscopy and a colonoscopy and found diverticulosis, abnormal outpouchings in the colon which are prone to bleeding. These outpouchings cannot be fixed with medication, therefore, a high-fiber diet was recommended. During that admission, Robert also was given a stress* *test which showed two areas of the heart that were receiving decreased blood flow under stress. A cardiac catheterization was recommended. Robert refused that test because he wanted to talk it over with Dr. A, his primary cardiologist who was not involved in the proposed treatment plan. He was discharged from the hospital on multiple medications and stool softeners to improve his bowel health.*

Dr. A saw no point in a catheterization because a patient must be able to take blood thinners in order to be considered for a catheterization and stenting. Stents in the heart require blood thinners to ensure that the stents stay open. Then even with stents in place, Robert would be prone to bleeding again when he was put on blood thinners because he still had untreated diverticulosis. With more bleeding, Robert would likely develop chest pain again even with the stents in place. Then, Dr. A believed that treating Robert would require healing the diverticulosis. She put him on a strict diet. She eliminated his animal products except fish and put him on a whole-grain, plant-based diet. Three months later, Robert had had no further rectal bleeding. His blood counts had risen significantly and he was no longer anemic. He had stopped taking his stool softeners and couldn't believe how regular his bowels were. He also no longer had any more chest pain. By six months later, Dr. A repeated a stress test and it was normal. Flow had normalized to all parts of his heart. Amazing.

THE KEY TO GOOD HEALTH IS SOMETIMES ELIMINATING, rather than adding. In order to subdue or treat our chronic illness we must minimize stresses on the body that cause inflammation. One of the most important stresses on the body is the food we take in which can have a lasting impact on the gut. Once we fix the gut, we begin to heal. Here, we will work on how we start the healing process.

ELIMINATION #1:
Remove Red Meat And Eggs from the diet for at least three months.

THE FIRST ELIMINATION that we would like people to work towards is elimination of meat and eggs. Start with the red meat. By red meat, we mean all beef, pork and venison in your diet, including hot dogs and sausages. Plan to completely rid your diet of these foods for at least three months. This time allows the gut to heal and the healthy gut flora to return. After the first six weeks of meat elimina-

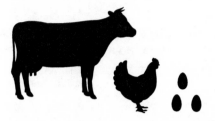

Figure 1:

Negative Health Efects of Meat and Eggs

Eating Red Meat and Eggs causes the gut to:

- **Produce TMAO** — which promotes plaque formation in the heart.

- **Elevate Saturated Fats** — linkrd to Heart Disease

- **Increase Production of lipopolysaccharide** — leading to dybiosis of the gut — causing leaky gut and inflammation

- **Elevate levels of salt** — linked to high blood pressure

- **increase nitrate levels** — endothelial dysfunction and insulin resistance

- **Elevate heterocyclic amines** — increase free radicals—increase risk of cancer

tion, we recommend giving up eggs. For some, this will be harder to give up than the red meat. Try to drop eggs completely for six weeks and then, if necessary, add them back once in a while as a treat. The gut needs that time to heal. Eventually, we would like you to stop eating poultry (turkey and chicken) as well. But this can come later. One step at a time.

Why is this elimination important? Recall that red meat and eggs cause the gut to produce TMAO which promotes plaque formation in the heart. We also know that a vegetarian diet and a high-fiber diet are associated with decreasing TMAO.[86] Other studies link red meat to heart disease due to the excess amount of saturated fat.[87] We know, too, that a high-fat diet which includes red meat causes production of lipopolysaccharide (LPS). Recall that LPS is responsible for dysbiosis and a leaky gut and is found in abundance in many chronic illness states. Then red meat is a trigger for inflammation.

What else do we know about the detrimental effects of meat? The salt in meat can be linked to high blood pressure. Nitrates, which are used as preservatives in meat, have been associated with poor dilation of the blood vessels (endothelial dysfunction)[88] and insulin resistance.[89] On the other hand, we know from Dean Ornish's early work that patients with heart disease who are put on a low-fat, plant-based diet saw less plaque in their heart arteries. Dr. Dean Ornish is a Harvard-trained physician who pioneered much of the early work on plant-based diet and heart disease. We also know from Caldwell Esselstyn's recent work at the Cleveland Clinic that adhering to a strictly plant-based diet can reduce plaque and increase blood flow to previously restricted areas.[90] *(Figure 1)*

Red meat is also associated with increased risk of many cancers.[91] Nitrate-derived metabolites, polycyclic aromatic hydrocarbons, and heterocyclic amines (HCAs)[92] are all possible carcinogens (cancer causing) and are found in red meat. Meat is cooked at high temperatures on the grill. When that meat darkens on the grill and is well done, HCAs are produced and appear to cause cancer. Even the excess iron in red meat may trigger some of these potential carcinogens.[93] Red meat is also thought to be a cause of oxidative stress which, as you may recall, is a stressor on the system that triggers formation of free radicals which are believed to be the starting point for cancer.[94]

The Tarahumara Indians of Mexico are known as "wellness warriors" because they are extremely active mountain runners and have virtually no coronary artery disease (heart disease clogs). Their diet is at least 90 percent beans and maize. Ninety-four percent of their protein comes from vegetable sources; only 6 percent is from animal sources. Of their fat intake, 33 percent is from vegetables and 67 percent comes from animals.[95] Most of their vegetable sources are corn and beans. Their cholesterol is derived from two eggs per week and rare courses of meat. The main source of calcium is the corn tortilla, made on limestone slabs so the tortillas absorb some of the calcium from the limestone.[96]

The data is compelling regarding this elimination. Red meat and eggs should be eliminated. We know this seems drastic. However, the impact of illness cannot be underestimated. These changes can happen and, if you want to be healthy, you must make them. Our recommendation is to start slowly, but deliberately.

What about fish and poultry? Eventually, we think we should eliminate at least all of our chicken. People are focused on chicken as a healthier option than red meat, but while it may be a slightly healthier option, it is not all that healthful. Chicken intake has grown significantly since the 1980s and the consumption of red meat has gone down by 30 percent, but chronic illnesses persist and continue to increase. Chicken is still too inflammatory for our bodies and should be significantly reduced or eliminated. We know this is tough love but as healthy-heart expert Dr. Caldwell Esselstyn says, "moderation kills." We must eliminate all of our red meat and chicken. Fish is the only meat for which we have substantial evidence that it lowers our risk of sudden death and coronary heart disease,[97, 98] probably due to its abundance of omega 3 fatty acids (more on fatty acids later). Data suggests eating two or more servings of fatty fish per week (mackerel, salmon, tuna) is associated with a decreased risk of heart disease.

Are we saying there is no room for an occasional meat dish? That's a difficult question. We know that eating meat is not good for our bodies. After three months of healing the microbiome can our bodies "tolerate" a little meat? Perhaps—it's hard to say for sure. Dr. A knows that with her chronic illness, she doesn't have room for "maybe." She feels that she has to be as close to perfect as possible because she doesn't want to get sick again. Can others who don't have a chronic illness still have some flexibility? Consider that heart disease is insidious. One-third of people with heart disease who die suddenly had no previous symptoms. We have to consider a patient's risk factors and determine what level of flexibility exists. *(Consider 1)*

At the same time, we would also say that everyone is doing their best. Eating less is always better than eating more. Do the best you can. Set goals and focus. You can do this. Consider the alternative: feeling bad, miserable even, and having a chronic illness. Isn't a healthy, meat-free diet worth a try?

> ## CONSIDER ❶
>
>  **Plan for three months of no meat or eggs which allows time for the gut to heal.** After that, is there room for an occasional meat or egg dish? Maybe, we don't know. Everyone's body will respond differently.

This is difficult for many people; they tell us they have eaten meat and potatoes their whole lives and can't imagine never eating them again. We always remind them that elimination is hard, but taking medications is hard too. What would you do if it meant you could stop taking medicine? What would you give up to live a longer, healthier life?

ELIMINATION #2:
Eliminate Dairy—All of it.

DAIRY REFERS TO MILK THAT COMES FROM COWS. Milk is obtained from cows on the farms. We then take that milk and we pasteurize it. Pasteurization is the process of heating something to high temperatures, then cooling it quickly; the goal is to kill microorganisms that develop with spoiled milk and give the product a longer shelf life.

The process works. It enables us to transfer milk from the farms to our grocery stores, so the milk will keep for ten days after opening. Before pasteurization, by the time dairy would get to the table it would be full of harmful bacteria and children were getting sick. So we started pasteurizing to avoid that bacteria formation, given the distance milk must travel and time that passes before we actually drink it.

With the pasteurization process, however, we not only remove the bacteria, but we also kill the enzymes that we need to break down milk in our bodies.[99] When the enzymes are destroyed, our bodies are not as equipped to process the milk. Many of us are sensitive to the milk and have a "milk allergy" or "milk sensitivity." We believe these dairy products trigger a leaky gut.[100] As dairy products enter the gut, the tight junctions break and the breakdown products of milk enter the bloodstream. Our immune system is activated and our bodies develop immune complexes that start attacking parts of the body. In some people, the joints are affected and we develop rheumatoid arthritis. In others, it is the pancreas islet cells that are attacked and we develop Type I diabetes. In others it is lupus, vitiligo (loss of pigment in the skin) or multiple sclerosis.

Milk digestion is enhanced by the lactase enzyme which breaks down lactose into D-glucose and D-galactose. In a study of mice,[101] the addition of D-galactose has been shown to induce signs of aging such as reduced cognitive and immune functions. At the same time in those mice, oxidative stress and chronic inflammation climbed. Remember, we believe it is these oxidative stresses that increase our risk for chronic illness. Negative changes in the products of genes (gene transcription factors) were also noted in the mice.[102] The idea that what we eat affects the activity of genes is an amazing concept. The amount of D-galactose given to the mice is the equivalent of 1-2 glasses of milk per day in humans. Consider then what impact that amount of milk could be having on

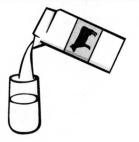

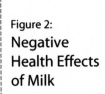

Figure 2:

Negative Health Effects of Milk

Consequences of Milk Sensitivity:

- **Leaky Gut** — leads to inflammation

- **D galactose ingestion which** — decreases cognitive function, decreases immune function, increases oxidative stress

- **Suggestion of potential increased fracture risk**

humans and consider milk's role in the process of aging. *(Figure 2)*

We know that chronic inflammation is a risk for heart disease and cancer. Inflammation is also a trigger for bone breakdown. Then suggesting that we humans drink more milk to decrease our fracture risk is a "conceivable contradiction." [103] There are many studies now that suggest a link between increased dairy and cardiovascular risk.[104],[105] In a follow-up to the these initial mouse studies, an extensive review was conducted to evaluate humans and milk intake, and one of the studies in the review evaluated people who drank more than three glasses of milk per day versus those who drank fewer than one glass per day. The research found a dose-dependent higher fracture and higher death rate in women who drank more milk. There was also a higher rate of death in men who drank more milk, though the fracture rate was not significantly different. Markers of inflammation and oxidative stress were also higher in those who drank more milk. [106]

In the 12-year Nurses' Health Study, nurses who drank more than two glasses of milk per day had no fewer fractures than those nurses consuming less than one glass of milk per week.[107] Interestingly, in that same Nurses' study, those who consumed greater amounts of calcium from dairy foods had higher fracture risk. That increased risk was not seen with calcium from non-dairy sources.[108]

This is really important. In other corroborating research, a meta-analysis of multiple larger trials showed there was no decrease in hip fractures with calcium supplementation.[109] This means that taking calcium supplements did not decrease rate of fractures. There may even have been a slightly higher fracture risk in people taking calcium supplements who didn't get adequate vitamin D.

Let's consider the occurrence of fractures around the world. In countries such as India, Japan and Peru, calcium intake is less than one-third of the daily recommended allowance (300mg per day), and the risk of fractures in those countries is extremely low. The countries with the highest fracture risks are actually those where people drank an abundance of milk, namely Norway, Sweden, Iceland, Denmark and the USA. These studies suggest that maybe drinking milk is not all it's cracked up to be! *(Consider 2)*

We also note that people with high sodium and high-protein diets absorb less calcium and excrete more calcium in their urine.[110] In the Nurses' Health Study, those nurses who took in more than 95 grams of protein per day were 20 percent more likely to fracture a bone than those who ingested less than 68 grams/day.[111] It is suspected that people with a diet lower in protein and sodium likely need less calcium in their diets. Protein from meat and eggs contains high concentrations of sulfate amino acids, which can cause calcium losses in the urine. Vegetarian diets are typically lower in protein than non-vegetarian

---

CONSIDER ❷

 Countries who drink less milk have fewer fractures

---

diets. Notably, however, both groups in the Nurses' Health Study exceeded the recommended daily allowance for protein (RDA). This may explain why people in countries where they typically eat less red meat and fat require less calcium.

We believe that building bones requires many components. We know that calcium is very important to bone development, but we don't know how much calcium we need, or the proper means of getting the calcium into our systems. Besides a diet rich in calcium, we know it is essential to have an abundance of vitamins D and K. In the Nurses' Health Study, researchers actually found an increase in fracture risk in women who consumed dairy sources for calcium versus those

---

CONSIDER ❸

 Spinach is rich in calcium but mostly calcium oxalate which may actually cause you to lose calcium in your urine. Eat spinach for iron and vitamins but not necessarily for calcium

---

who consumed non-dairy sources of calcium *(Figure 3)*.

Calcium comes from many non-dairy sources, including broccoli,

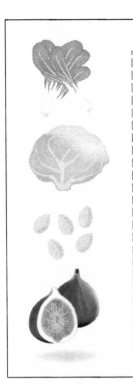

Figure 3:
Nondairy Sources of Calcium.

- **Kale** — ½ cup (90 mg)

- **Collard Greens** — ½ cup (178 mg)

- **Turnip Greens** — 6 oz (220 mg)

- **Bok Choy** — ½ cup (190 mg)

- **Almonds** — 3 oz (210 mg)

- **Sesame Seeds** — 1 tbsp (51 mg)

- **Blackstrap Molasses** — 1 tbsp (172 mg)

- **Chia Seeds** — 1.5 oz (300 mg)

- **Figs** — 5 whole (135 mg)

kale, collard greens, turnip greens (6 ounces contain 220mg calcium), bok choy, almonds (3 ounces have 210 mg), sunflower seeds, tahini, dried beans and blackstrap molasses. Flax seeds and sesame seeds are two more great sources of calcium.[112] Calcium in low-oxalate vegetables such as kale is readily absorbed, so they are viable options for calcium intake in a plant-based diet.[113] *(Consider 3)*

VITAMIN D

VITAMIN D IS ALSO VERY IMPORTANT in bone health. It helps us to absorb calcium and not lose it when we urinate. Vitamin D is produced by the skin when we are exposed to sunlight. However, winter sun is not strong enough in regions above 40 degrees latitude (north of Philadelphia and San Francisco) to aid in converting vitamin D to its active form. Sunscreens, while effective for preventing sun damage, inhibit the production of vitamin D. Therefore, many of us are vitamin D deficient, regardless of whether we drink milk or not. Cow's milk does NOT have vitamin D in it, so we fortify it with vitamin D. Similarly, almond milk also is fortified with vitamin D. We have data to suggest that vitamin D (700-800 IU) is a daily dose that lowers the risk of hip fracture.[114] This is not the same for children and the childrens' dosing should be discussed.

VITAMIN K

VITAMIN K IS ANOTHER IMPORTANT VITAMIN for bone health. Data shows that taking in less than 110 micrograms of vitamin K can increase your fracture risk. In a study of nurses, those who ate a serving of greens every day experienced only half the fractures as those who ate just one serving per week.[115] The Framingham heart study corroborated this idea.[116] Broccoli, kale, brussel sprouts and collard greens are good sources of vitamin K.

Other substances in our diets may also raise our risk of osteoporosis. Excess coffee/caffeine may increase our kidneys' removal of calcium from our bloodstream. In the Framingham osteoporosis study, older women who drank caffeinated soda had a higher incidence of fractures than those who did not.

The bottom line: We have no data to suggest that dairy is needed to lower our risk of osteoporosis. We do need calcium, but we don't need much. We also need vitamins D and K to help the calcium build bone density. The goal should be to eat calcium-rich, nondairy products. Guidelines recommend 1000 mg of calcium below the age of 50 years and 1200mg in postmenopausal women. However, there is no scientific data to confirm that drinking cow's milk is better than the alternatives. We need to focus on the a diet with lots of calcium rich greens (also rich in vitamin K) and an adequate dose of vitamin D daily.

WHAT ABOUT MILK AND CANCER?

STUDIES SUGGEST A CORRELATION between milk intake and bladder and prostate cancer, as well as a potential link with colon cancer.[117] There are connections between galactose and ovarian cancer. This association was found in women who drank more than three glasses of milk per day.[118] In a Harvard study of male professionals, men who drank more than two glasses of milk per day were at an increased risk of prostate cancer compared to those who did not drink milk.[119] In another study, men who consumed more than 2000 mg of calcium suffered almost double the rate of fatal prostate cancer than those who did not. There has been much speculation about the increased risks of reproductive cancers from drinking milk produced from cows that were injected with different hormones to produce excess milk.[120]

Recent studies have also linked milk to an increase in acne, which may be related to the hormones in milk.[121]

T. Colin Campbell, author of The China Study, also feels that over-consumption of animal-based proteins can be detrimental to health. He specifically conducted rat and mice studies, which showed that a 20-percent casein (milk protein) diet promoted liver cancer in the animals, and when the animals were fed a reduced casein diet of 5 percent, their tumor growth was reduced. Even when the diet was switched from high to low casein, the results were the same—reduced casein resulted in less tumor growth. Animals that consumed a diet containing 20 percent casein were all dead at 100 weeks.[122] Even though these studies are based on rats and mice, they point to a possible concern about consuming too much casein.

WHAT ABOUT MILK AND AUTOIMMUNE DISEASE?

MILK HAS BEEN LINKED TO inflammation and oxidative stress.[123] How milk triggers inflammation is not entirely clear. However, it is likely through the leaky gut (see chapter 6). In some people, milk is like gluten, triggering breakdown of the tight junction and allowing food products to enter the bloodstream. These food products prompt an attack from our gut defense system, bringing on a full inflammatory response: body on fire. Dr. A believes strongly that dairy triggered her leaky gut and caused the autoimmune reaction of her disease. Eliminating milk products healed her.

WHAT ABOUT YOGURT AND SOUR MILK?

IT IS IMPORTANT TO NOTE THAT IN STUDIES, the same level of inflammation was not noted when people drank sour milk or ate yogurt. In fact, a negative relationship was found; i.e. sour milk and yogurt did not increase inflammation and may actually decrease inflammation.[124] These findings may be related to the fact that there is significantly lower to no lactose and galactose in these fermented products and they may also have probiotic antioxidant and anti-inflammatory benefits.[125] More study is required on yogurt and fermented milk products. Likely, they do not have the same effect on the body as regular milk products. If you have to choose milk products, these are the ones to choose.

MILK IN OUR DAILY LIFE

THERE IS A GREAT DEAL OF DATA that suggests that people live shorter lives when they drink milk and most notably, they do NOT have fewer fractures. The popular conception that milk helps build strong bones needs to be reconsidered and modified. Dr. A's children have been told that they're eating a bad diet because it does not have milk in it. If they buy a school lunch, they are required to take milk. When we look at the healthy school meal, it always includes milk. Are we teaching our kids the right thing?

The American diet has butter and cheese in almost everything. If you get a side of black beans at a Mexican restaurant, there is always a sprinkle of Cheddar cheese on it. If you get a salad, you usually get a sprinkle of mozzarella or Parmesan. Pasta sauces and soups have cream in them. This elimination is hard, no question, and takes education and effort. However, once you feel better, your sacrifice will will be worth it.

Figure 4:
**Alternatives
to Cow's Milk**

- **soy milk and yogurt**
- **almond milk and yogurt**
- **coconut milk and yogurt**
- **cashew cream**
- **nut cheeses**

So, start by removing the milk from the house. Buy almond or soy milk instead; there are many brands on the market these days, including unsweetened and unflavored options. Try to drink the ones in the refrigerated section because they contain fewer additives. You can even buy chocolate almond milk, which is delicious.

Instead of butter, which is made with cow's milk, switch to a plant-based margarine. You won't notice the difference. You also can find coconut, soy and almond milk yogurts.

Get rid of your cheese and replace it with soy cheese alternatives. These options don't taste as good as real cheese, but some people like them in transition. Soy cheese alternatives have the same texture as real cheese, but they don't melt in the same way and they taste different. Personally, Dr. A would rather not eat cheese now at all. It seems strange to her to that she doesn't miss it when she was so addicted to dairy for so long. You will get there, too! *(Figure 4, Consider 4)*

Success comes with baby steps. Don't add cheese to your salads and eat bread without butter. Use almond or soy milk in your tea or morning coffee. Make oatmeal with water instead of milk. Try eating a pizza with good, fresh dough, tasty sauce and a few vegetables. One of our favorite pizzas is black olives and pepperoncini on pizza. You can make an amazing cream for dressings and "cheesy" cream sauces with blended cashews and nutritional yeast. There are so many options available, you will be surprised.

People often say they don't enjoy the texture or taste of certain foods. As we tell our kids, you sometimes have to try things 10 times before you like them. We remember when our kids first started eating salads. They complained and complained. Six months later, Dr. A's kids love spinach. How does that happen? We all change. Our tastes change. We adapt. We do what is necessary to be healthy, and when our bodies feel better because we're eating different foods, it is a game changer.

> **CONSIDER ❹**
>
> √ **Next time you are ordering pizza at a restaurant or even take out, ask them to hold the cheese.** Try it, you might be surprised and every place we have ever eaten will make this for you

ARE WE GETTING ENOUGH PROTEIN?

PEOPLE OFTEN BECOME highly concerned about getting sufficient protein and calcium in a diet that includes no dairy, eggs or meat. This is what we are asked the most: how will I get my protein on such a diet? For those just starting their transitions and still eating chicken and fish, protein sources are evident. For those of us who have taken it to the next level and completely eliminated all animal products, we promise you that you will get enough protein! People don't become protein deficient anymore unless they are truly starving. Some of the best athletes in the world eat completely plant-based diets. Dr. A did her first triathlon after going completely plant-based. You will have plenty of energy and in fact, probably will have more with all the plant-based foods and as we teach you to eat minimally processed, no added sugar foods.

ELIMINATE #3: PROCESSED FOODS

PROCESSED FOODS ARE THOSE THAT HAVE BEEN ALTERED from their natural state. This refers to any food that has been canned, frozen, dehydrated, pasteurized or changed by other means.

IS PROCESSING A BAD THING?

OfTEN, WE PROCESS FOODS to make them last longer by canning, freezing or dehydrating them. That is not necessarily a bad thing. It allows for many conveniences. We pasteurize food to kill harmful bacteria so it can last longer on our shelves. However, pasteurization often kills healthy enzymes as well. Many processed foods include an abundance of saturated fats, oils, and salt. Oily, fried and fatty products last longer. The problem is that excess fats and oils put us at risk for cardiovascular disease, and excess sodium increases risk of high blood pressure.

We also process foods by adding preservatives to make them last longer. Sometimes we use sodium to preserve foods, such as with our deli meats, and at other times we use artificial preservatives. Preservatives and artificial flavors are often highly inflammatory, which starts the spiral toward chronic illness. Many foods also contain high fructose corn syrup, an artificial sweetener. Corn syrup was introduced into the food market decades ago because sugar was too expensive. We had an abundance of corn, and corn syrup was easy to make and could be done without significant expense. Now, corn syrup is in a huge percentage of products in the United States—even found in ketchup! The problem with high fructose corn syrup is that it is an unnatural sweetener and, therefore, it is inflammatory. It blocks our natural desire to stop eating and prevents us from feeling full (recall leptin resistance). We don't feel satiated as easily when we eat high fructose corn syrup, therefore we are more likely to overeat and become obese.

Consider how much of our food comes in a bag or lasts on the shelf for weeks on end. Food shouldn't last that long. It should go bad, and food without excess processing and preservatives will. There is no question that we need to preserve foods to get through harsh winters and travel. Canning and dehydrating are great options for this.

Another form of processing is refined foods. Often food we buy has gone from being whole-grain to a thin remnant of its former self. Consider oatmeal for a second. Whole grain oats are large and thick, at least 1-2 mm thick. When you buy instant oatmeal, the oats are 0.1 mm thick. They have been shaved down to become more palatable but all of the fiber benefits are gone. Our breads are similar. Our wheat has been thinned and broken down and then made into bread. This makes the bread go down smoothly but we have lost all the benefits of the product. This is what has given bread a bad name. Refined products have minimal fiber and little nutritional value. We want our food to have bulk. It is good for digestion and good for increasing density of food in our stomachs and for making us feel full.

When we first started our eliminating processed foods, we began by saying we wouldn't eat food that was sold in a bag. That is difficult these days when half the food in the grocery store is bagged. We started buying our bread in the bakery section of the supermarket, where the breads often don't have artificial pre-servatives in them. We now go grocery shopping a few times a week. We buy fresh food and eat it for a few days until we finish it. Then we go back for more. People often say they are too busy to go to the grocery store more than once per week, but we find that life is simpler now. We buy fresh food, cook and enjoy it. The flavors that come from fresh foods are one-of-a-kind.

A NOTE ON CANNED FOODS

CANNED FOODS are preserved but very practical, especially in the winter. While we encourage eating fresh, that is not always possible. You can buy canned foods, such as beans and vegetables that have only salt in them as a preservative. Look for these. Wash the beans thoroughly which removes about one-third of the sodium.

> **CONSIDER ❺**
>
> √ **Canned foods are not the enemy. Ideally, we don't eat canned vegetables and eat them fresh. Canned beans are very useful in a busy household. Canned foods do have salt in them as a preservative which is the negative.** Salt restriction is most important in patients with heart failure and some restriction is necessary with high blood pressure. Most people though can tolerate canned beans without difficulty. Rinse them thoroughly and that will remove about 1/3 of the salt

Another great option for beans and legumes are dried, dehydrated beans. There are no preservatives in these. You do have to plan those meals beforehand, though, because dried beans and legumes often require soaking for 24 hours before you cook them. Slow cookers and pressure cookers, however, are more efficient. *(Consider 5)*

SUGARS: OUR NEWEST ADDICTION

PROCESSED SWEETENERS ARE THE MOST COMMON food additives worldwide. In 2009, Americans consumed an average of more than 130 pounds of processed sweeteners a year![126] That translates to an av-

Figure 5:
Alternatives
to Artificial Sweeteners

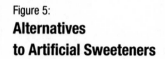

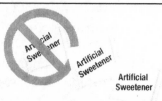

Artificial
Sweetener

Don't use artificial sweeteners. They don't make you lose weight and likely make you gain weight. They are also inflammatory.

First try your coffee/tea without any sugar at all! You will get used to it over time. Sugar is a drug and with time and slow weaning, you won't miss it.

Before you get to the "no added sugar" option: try these options while you wean:

- **Dates:** great in cooking, super sweet
- **Blueberries:** great in cooking, super sweet
- **Applesauce**
- **Cane sugar** (regular sugar)
- **Honey**

The Bottom Line — We would rather you eat sugar than an artificial sweetener.

erage of one-third of a pound (about 5.7 ounces, 160 grams, or 36 teaspoons) of processed sweeteners each day, per person. This consumption is almost seven times the American Heart Association guidelines of 24 grams of processed sugar per day for women (approximately 6 teaspoons, which is a little less than 1 ounce) and more than four times the 36 grams per day recommended for men (about 9 teaspoons).[127] For a very simple example, one 12-ounce soda contains an average of about 40 grams of added sugars, well in excess of the recommended daily sugar intake.

Artificial sweeteners exist because they are supposedly low-calorie alternatives to sugar. People think that when they drink their coffee with artificial sweeteners, they won't gain weight. But is that true? In one population-based study, 474 people were followed for almost 10 years. Those participants who drank diet soda had a 70-percent higher increase in waist circumference than non-diet soda consumers. Those who drank two or more diet sodas per day reported a shocking 500-percent increase in waist circumference over non-diet soda consumers![128]

Another study was done on rats which were fed the artificial sweetener, aspartame; they subsequently showed an increase in blood glucose without a decrease in insulin-producing cells, suggesting insulin resistance. This study suggested that drinking diet soda could be a risk for developing diabetes.[129]

A more recent study in 2013 showed that diet drinks contribute to obesity.[130] A recent article in Nature[131] linked artificial sweeteners with dysbiosis (disruption of the microbiome) and increased insulin resistance (prediabetes). These studies show that artificial sweeteners are not better and are likely, worse. We do not believe in diet drinks. They worsen the obesity problem and should be completely avoided. We are only fooling ourselves if we drink them. *(Figure 5)*

Most processed foods are bad for us. Cookies and cakes sit on the store shelf for weeks full of preservatives so that they don't get hard. Artificial sweeteners are added into our foods so they will have "zero calories." Artificial sweeteners are chemicals and they make us sick. Learn to read labels and don't eat processed foods. Consider that if you want to eat cookies, make them yourself. Buy fresh ingredients and you won't go wrong. Make pumpkin bread and cornbread using a mix but just change the egg to applesauce with baking powder (1 egg=4 oz. applesauce and 1 tsp. of baking powder) and cow's milk to coconut milk. You will need less oil when you use applesauce. If you want pizza, make the dough yourself and use red sauce with an abundance of vegetables.Skip the cheese! Yum. *(Figure 6—see page 89)*

WHAT OTHER HARMFUL FOODS DO WE EAT?

TOO MANY OF US HAVE ABSOLUTELY NO IDEA what is in our food. Often we see words on the ingredient lists that we've never heard of, but we just accept that they are safe to eat. Most of what we eat comes in a package and we have no contact with the source of our food.

Reading the ingredient list can be intimidating, so most people don't even bother looking at it. We hope that after reading the information presented here, you will become a real nutrition label detective, reading and evaluating all of the ingredients in any packaged food before you purchase it. Part of the problem is that we have lost that connection with our food. Many city dwellers in America today haven't seen how fresh food is grown. We often don't know how foods grow in their native climates. Most of us definitely do not grow our own. Home-cooked meals made with fresh ingredients are rarities in many households. We rely on packaged foods, restaurant meals and "fast food."

We also expect the government and food industry to protect us from potentially harmful ingredients. But are they really protecting us? In eating mostly processed foods, we are regularly exposed to "new" food products that are not natural to the human body, including:

- genetically modified organisms (GMOs)
- artificial colorings and flavorings
- high fructose corn syrup and artificial sweeteners
- processed fats, including hydrogenated oils and even trans-fats
- naturally occurring saturated fats from animals often eating GMO feed
- fertilizers and pesticides
- over-processed "refined" grains
- animal products that can contain drugs, including antibiotics and growth hormones

GENETICALLY MODIFIED ORGANISMS (GMOS)

GMOs are plants or animals that have been genetically altered by inserting genes from foreign bacteria, viruses, insects, and other sources into the DNA of the host plant or animal. Originally introduced into our food supply in the 1990s, GMOs in plants typically are genetic modifications that allow the plant to either withstand heavy applications of pesticides, or actually produce pesticides in the plant itself. The inserted genes are from living organisms that have different DNA than the original food or animal. There has been no requirement by the government for any testing to prove the safety of GM foods for human consumption. We have only the manufacturer's claim that GM foods are safe for human consumption. In the United States we currently have no labeling laws requiring food manufacturers to label GM foods, so you do not even know when you are consuming a genetically altered product and the majority of corn and soy produced in America are genetically modified.

The main upside to GMO crops is that we have created a more durable product that can potentially increase the yield of food. However, there is significant concern that genetically altering food affects how our bodies deal with it, creating inflammation and triggering chronic illness. A variety of animal studies implicate GMOs as potential health hazards, but very few human studies have been completed. One human

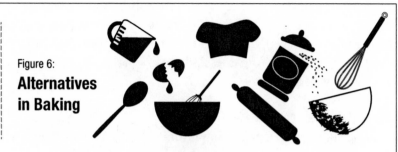

Figure 6:
Alternatives in Baking

EGG ALTERNATIVES

1. **Tofu-can be used as a "egg" scramble.**
   1/4 cup of puréed tofu = 1 egg

2. **Applesauce** — used in baking,
   1/4 cup applesauce with 1 teaspoon of baking powder = 1 egg

3. **Potato starch** — 2 tbsp potato starch = 1 egg

4. **Prunes** — 1/4 cup pureed prunes = 1 egg

5. **Flax seeds** — need to soak and becomes good binder:
   1 tbsp ground flax with 3 tbsp water, leave to soak for 5 minutes

6. **Banana** — 1/2 banana = 1 egg

DAIRY ALTERNATIVES

1. **Consider almond or soy milk**

2. **Soy cheese alternatives**

3. **Blended cashews make a nice cream salad dressing or creamy cheese with nutritional yeast**

4. **Soy or coconut milk yogurts**

study, completed in Canada in 2011, discovered some of the pesticides associated with GM foods were found in the blood of both pregnant and non-pregnant women in Canada.[132] This is concerning, but the true impact on the body is not known.

The American Academy of Environmental Medicine suggested to its members in 2008 that they educate their patients about the potential health dangers of GMOs.[133]   Overall, we recommend trying to avoid genetically modified foods. This can be done by choosing organic foods. The most common genetically modified foods are corn, soybeans, canola and cottonseed oils. Tomatoes and potatoes are also often genetically modified as well as papaya.

OTHER THINGS TO CONSIDER:

DAIRY PRODUCTS often come from cows treated with genetically engineered hormones and antibiotics.

Many cereals and breakfast bars contain genetically modified ingredients.

Read all labels on any packaged foods before you purchase them. Frozen dinners, soups, salad dressings, snack foods, candy, chocolates, sodas, juices and condiments may contain many GMO ingredients (look on the label for the words corn, soy, canola and cottonseed and avoid those products).

Consider that the most important thing we can do to heal is elimination. ▪

YOUR PRESCRIPTION:

Commit To Elimination

Know you can do this. Elimination will cleanse your body and heal your microbiome.

- **Eliminate red meat, eggs and dairy** for at least three months.

- **Eliminate highly processed foods.** Think natural.

- **Eat fresh**.

- **Go to the grocery store** a few times per week.

- **Go to a bakery** for your bread.

- **If you want to eat cookies**, bake them yourselves.

CHAPTER 8:

SUPER FOODS: Greens, Beans, Carbs, Oh My!

Adding back

WHEN DR. A WAS YOUNGER, she constantly battled her weight. She always felt overweight and worried. She ate diet bars and drank diet Coke. She starved herself at times and weighed herself at least once a day and usually would feel disappointed. We know the feeling when nothing fits, or the feeling of not wanting to take your shirt off at the swimming pool to show off your body. After Dr. A had her three children and got so sick, she learned how to eat. Dr. A and Dr. R don't eat any weight-reducing foods. They just eat healthily and feel great.

In the last chapter, we spent a lot of time talking about which foods to take out of the diet—toxins—to allow for gut healing. As with everything, we have to balance that by adding back resources for the body—foods that replenish and restore. This chapter will focus on replenishment of resources and is as important as what we eliminate.

ADD BACK FRUITS AND VEGETABLES

THE IMPORTANCE OF FRUITS AND VEGETABLES has been purported for centuries. Fruits contain vitamins A and C as well as potassium. Vegetables give us an abundance of fiber, vitamins A and C, iron, magnesium, calcium and potassium. They even have protein. Fruits and vegetables are rich in phytonutrients (plant nutrients) and plant sterols (discussed previously). These phytonutrients have been shown in many trials to be beneficial. In times of acute stress, phytonutrients activate stress signals, which are important in cell defense.[134]

Then, phytonutrients arm us with defenses against damage and illness. Phytonutrients are also antioxidants. You may recall that oxidation occurs with prolonged distress and triggers free radicals, which are cancer promoting and increase inflammation. The antioxidant effect of phytonutrients, then, is to decrease inflammation.

Phytonutrients can be broken down into important components such as carotenoids, flavonoids, resveratrol and phytoestrogens. The more brightly colored the fruits and vegetables, the more abundant they are in these components. Different vegetables have different phytonutrients in them which is why people often say to 'eat the rainbow' *(Figure 1)*. Red vegetables such as tomatoes are known for lycopene which is believed to lower men's risk of prostate cancer.[136] Recent data suggests it may also reduce our risk of strokes.[137] Orange fruits and vegetables such as oranges and pumpkins have beta carotene among other components. Beta-carotene may bring added benefits because it is converted to vitamin A. Beta-carotenoids such as lutein and zeaxanthin are found in most vegetables and in abundance in our green leafy vegetables.

These vitamin A precursors are also found in abundance in our eyes and appear to protect against eye diseases.[138] Blue colored fruits such as grapes, red wine and blueberries are rich in flavonoids such as reservatrol which is a potent antioxidant and appear to have a role in dilating (opening up) our blood vessels and may help with decreasing risk of heart disease. [139,140,141] It also has a potential anti-aging effect as shown in mice studies. Human studies, however, are inconclusive.[142] Since not all fruits and vegetables possess all phytonutrients, it is important to eat a variety of colors to ensure you are getting all of the health benefits.

HOW MUCH IS ENOUGH?

OVER THE CENTURIES, the benefits of fruits and vegetables have long been purported. However, it has been unclear how many is really enough. In 1990, the World Health Organization decided to quantify a recommended amount. At that time, they recommended a minimum intake of 400 grams of fruits and vegetables per day to decrease the risk of cardiovascular disease and cancer.[142] Shortly after, the idea of five servings of fruits and vegetables per day was adopted by the United Kingdom and subsequently by France and Germany. The United States then adopted a "more is better" stance and it became a fairly widespread concept that fruits and vegetables should be encouraged.

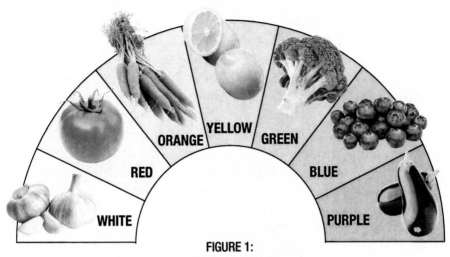

FIGURE 1:

THE FOOD RAINBOW
Build your meals around your colors:

WHITE: allicin: garlic, onions, leeks, chives

RED: lycopene: tomatoes, guava, watermelon

ORANGE: beta carotene: carrots, pumpkins

YELLOW: beta carotene, flavonoids: oranges and lemons

GREEN: lutein, folic acid: kale, spinach, mustard greens, broccoli, brussel sprouts

BLUE: flavonoids: grapes, red wine, blueberries, beets

PURPLE: phenols: eggplant, dried raisins, plums

But there has been much debate about how effective fruits and vegetables are in combating chronic illness. Their role in reducing cardiovascular illness has been shown in multiple meta-analyses[143] and is quite compelling but whether they lower cancer risk has been less clear. In 2013, a study was published that showed when we eat more fruits and vegetables, we live longer. This relationship was most notable in relation to reduction in cardiovascular deaths (heart disease). In this same study, the relationship was more compelling in

 CONSIDER ❶

When we eat more fruits and vegetables, we live longer! Don't think so much about which fruit or vegetable is better, all are good. Eat them often and much.

raw vegetables than cooked.[144] (*Consider 1*).

A 2014 British analysis[145] showed a significant survival benefit for those eating one to three servings of fruits and vegetables versus less than one serving per day. However, the survival benefit was highest in those who ate more than seven servings per day. Further, this study showed that the benefits were most notable with higher intake of different varieties of vegetables, salads, fresh fruit and dried fruit. Canned and frozen fruit consumption also conferred a survival benefit. In this study, however, canned and frozen fruits were lumped together and therefore, the benefit of each individually could not be assessed. Of note, however, canned and dried fruit often have a significantly higher sugar content than frozen fruits.

While some studies suggest vegetables are more important in overall survival, other studies have shown that fruits are better.[146] We feel there is enough data to suggest that they are both good. People often ask which fruits and vegetables are of the most benefit. We tell people that it doesn't matter. They are all good. However, the ratio likely should be closer to two vegetables per one fruit. Remember, fruits have more simple sugars (fructose) which can be an issue in patients with diabetes.

Overall, fruits and vegetables are great when eaten raw. However, there are some vegetables that are more nutritionally potent when they are cooked. It's hard to remember all of the details sometimes such as which vegetables are more potent when cooked. We try to keep it simple and just tell people to eat as many colors as they can throughout the day: raw, cooked, frozen, whatever. The bottom line is eating more than seven servings per day of fruits and vegetables lowers heart disease risk, has a role in decreasing cancer, and all-cause mortality.

Many people feel overwhelmed when they consider that they have to eat seven servings of fruits and vegetables every day. People often ask how to incorporate them into their meals. In the morning, Dr. A often has a banana and two pieces of toast with hummus. She eats fresh bread from the bakery, which has minimal sugar and no preservatives. Then around 10am, she eats 20-30 baby carrots, usually with hummus again. For lunch, she often eats a huge spinach or kale salad with an abundance of vegetables and seeds. Around 3pm, she might have an apple. For dinner, she will often eat a veggie burger with steamed broccoli, or a bowl of rice and lentils with that same steamed broccoli or sautéed bok choy. For dessert, an orange (or nothing at all) is enough.

When you think it through, it can be easy to get seven to 10 servings of vegetables per day!

Bottom line is to try for diversity and remember to eat all of the colorful vegetables—don't limit yourself. For instance, red and yellow peppers are full of phytonutrients. Spinach is full of iron but doesn't provide calcium and may even leach calcium you've just eaten from other sources. Turnip greens, mustard greens, bok choy and kale, among others, have plenty of calcium, so vary it up and eat all the colorful vegetables, all of the time. *(Consider 2)*

> **CONSIDER ❷**
>
> √ When you are thinking about your fruits and vegetables for the day, you don't have to remember what fruit or vegetable has what in it. Just remember to eat a variety of colors. Eat greens, reds, oranges, blues and purples. Don't get stuck on just one color, you won't get the full benefits.

Regarding fruit, we eat these in abundance as well. Fresh fruit is likely the most potent, so try to eat whole fruits. Think about pomegranates, too, which are full of antioxidants and potentially decrease inflammation and stressors in your body. Try to vary your fruits as well because they all offer such different nutrients—but eat them often and in large quantities and you will not go wrong. Citrus has vitamin C. Berries are abundant in antioxidants. Bananas are rich in potassium.

People with diabetes often tell us their doctors say they cannot eat fruits. But then, those same patients eat refined breads and cookies because they want something sweet and they're hungry. We would take any fruit over that option, any day of the week. Most often, the fruit is not the problem for people with diabetes; usually everything else in the diet is the culprit.

A FEW WORDS ABOUT KALE

KALE HAS RECEIVED A LOT OF PRESS LATELY as the wonder vegetable, a super food. It really is an amazing vegetable. It contains an abundance of vitamin A, potassium and magnesium. It also has iron, calcium and protein and a bounty of B vitamins, including folate which helps in brain development. Kale also contains fiber, which is good for lowering cholesterol levels, as well as alpha linoleic acid (ALA), a precursor to omega-3 fatty acids. ALA also has been shown to decrease the risk of heart disease.[147] Omega-3 fatty acids are important in decreasing inflammation and should be part of the daily diet. Kale also has lutein which helps to prevent macular degeneration. We try to eat kale at least three times per week. You can choose from three different types of kale: lacinato, green and red kale. They are all good! Eat them all. You can take the stems out of the lacinato kale (they are hard to eat) and add the stems to a soup or broth.

JUICES AND SHAKES

WE OFTEN HEAR QUESTIONS about juicing and shakes. Whole fruits and vegetables, rather than juices, are absolutely the best and should be encouraged. In their liquid form, as with juicing, all of the essential fibers are removed from the food. You have nothing to chew on to stimulate your gut enzymes, which are essential for good digestion. When we juice, we get the vitamins and lots of sugar, without those fibers. When we eat the food raw, we have so much more. If you really like to drink juice, drink small amounts and think about pomegranate juice which has many potent antioxidants.

What about shakes? We do use a super blender on occasion. When you use these super blenders, the fruits and vegetables are broken down but the fibers stay inside the drink. It is good that the fibers are still inside but probably not as good as the whole food because the fibers are broken up. When you eat the whole food you have to chew, which activates the digestive enzymes. The whole fibers bring down your cholesterol levels and decrease inflammation. At the end of the day, shakes are good because they are quick and allow a quick way to get in a lot of vegetables at once. Are whole fruits and vegetables even a little better? Sure! Do the best you can. If shakes work, go for it.

THE IMPORTANCE OF THE CARBOHYDRATE: LEGUMES AND BEANS

CARBOHYDRATES (CARBS) HAVE GOTTEN A BAD RAP lately, and we want to give you our two cents about the underappreciated carbohydrate. So many diets tell us to avoid carbohydrates because they are the reason we gain weight. This concept is the foundation for many "low carb" or "no carb" diets which often focus on counting carbs to keep our weight down. We don't believe in these diets and counting carbs. Without carbs, we lose so many essential nutrients and fiber. Carbs also allow us to feel full. The nutrients in carbohydrates are es-

FIGURE 2:
A LEGUMES SAMPLER
Legumes are low glycemic and high in fiber, resistant starches

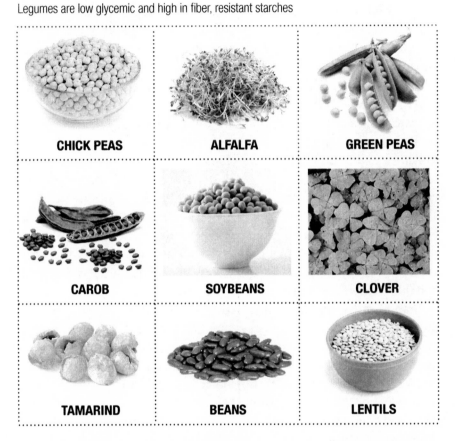

CHICK PEAS	ALFALFA	GREEN PEAS
CAROB	SOYBEANS	CLOVER
TAMARIND	BEANS	LENTILS

sential because they provide us with the energy for day-to-day living. They give us our energy to get up and go. People gain weight when they eat carbs mostly because the carbs they are eating are refined and highly processed, not the whole-grain carbohydrates we should be eating. When you eat whole-grain carbs, your body will tell you when to stop eating. You will feel full, contented and full of energy.

Let's talk about the chemistry a bit. Carbohydrates can be broken into complex carbohydrates and simple carbohydrates. The simple carbs are mostly sugars. They are good for short bursts of energy but have no lasting effect. The more complex the structure, the longer it takes to break it down, which causes less rise in blood glucose (blood sugar) levels. This is the concept of the glycemic index. Foods that have a low glycemic index are more complex in structure—more whole-grain—and take longer to break down and, thus, raise your blood glucose to only a low level. Those foods high on the glycemic index, such as candy, chips, cookies and other processed foods are simple sugars and break down easily. Because low-glycemic index foods take longer to break down, they bring about a feeling of satiety faster than high-glycemic foods, and less drastic boosts in blood sugar levels.

It is not only a food's "ranking" on the glycemic index that's important, though. Food in its natural form provides a lot of fiber. Beans are carbohydrates but are full of fiber and water so they take longer to break down. Because they take time to break down, they don't cause the quick highs and lows that simple sugars such as refined breads and sodas can cause; they steadily break down over time. These complex carbohydrates give us a measured amount of energy at all times. It gets a little confusing when we look at pasta. Pasta is a low-glycemic food, which is good, but it has minimal fiber. On the other hand, it is better than eating candy and cookies, which have a high glycemic index without any fiber, therefore, are processed moderately quickly. Pasta is good and filling but doesn't have the fiber we need.

Grapes and fruits are considered "simple" carbohydrates because they are primarily sugar, but they are good for us because they also provide us with fibrous strands and bulk. As you can see, not all simple carbohydrates are a problem. It is what we do to the foods, the processing. When we process them, they become simple and they lose their fiber: two negatives. Studies show that increased fiber is associated with decreased heart disease.[148] Studies also show that whole grains are better than simple/refined grains.[149]

The foundational complex carbohydrates are legumes, which come from plants. They have a low glycemic index and are high in fiber. (*Figure 2*) Examples of legumes are alfalfa, clover, lentils, peas (green peas and chick peas), beans, carob, soybeans, peanuts and tamarind. Beans of any kind are excellent food choices. Consider kidney beans, black beans, navy beans, and pinto beans, and they are all amazing! There are so many vital ingredients in these legumes. They are rich in protein and high in potassium. Many contain a significant amount of magnesium and iron. Some legumes also provide a little calcium, but not a significant amount.

Legumes also contain resistant starches. When resistant starches reach the colon, they ferment and form short-chain fatty acids such as butyrate. Butyrate production appears to be important in maintaining colonic health and lowering our risk of chronic illness. Butyrate increases leptin production which, you recall, is our satiety hormone—so legumes make us feel full! Research suggests that butyrate also is vital in lowering insulin resistance, risk of stroke and high cholesterol. It also appears related to a diminishing risk of cancer.[150] Legumes are truly amazing foods!

Another way to look at foods is based on their caloric density. Jeff Novick at the McDougall Center in Santa Rosa, California is a huge proponent of this approach to food. Think of caloric density as the amount of calories per ounce of food. Water and fiber in food will lower its calorie density, while fat and oil increase it. Studies show that overall, people eat about the same amount of food every day, but if you eat, say, half a pound of calorie-dense food such as glazed donuts, you'll take in many more calories than if you eat half a pound of lettuce, which has very little calorie density.

We also need water and fiber in foods to increase satiety. Consider that chili is high in caloric density, but if you add vegetables to chili its density

FIGURE 3:

Examples of Low Density and High Density Meals

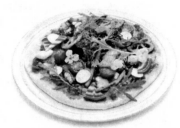

Low Calorie Density Meal (GOOD)

- 12 oz water
- Kale salad with hummus
- Veggie pizza without cheese
- Or bowl of rice and beans with sprouts, onions, tomatoes and spinach
- Low calorie density snack: raw veggies and hummus

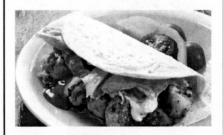

High Density Meal (NOT GOOD)

- Juice
- Beef taco with shredded cheese, sour cream
- Grilled chicken, beans, sour cream in burrito
- High calorie dense snack: granola bar or cheese stick

will be less because vegetables are full of fiber and water. Studies show that people who eat lower caloric-density foods can eat more food by weight and still take in fewer calories than those who eat high-fat, high-caloric density foods.[151] In other words, you don't have to re-strict your portions if you eat less calorie-dense. You will also feel full because you haven't restricted your portion. The Centers for Disease Control (CDC)[152] points out that people who eat lower caloric density foods can consume fewer calories without changing how much they eat. Many studies show that when people eat foods with low caloric density, they lose weight without changing the amount they eat, and they feel satiated.[153,154] (Consider 3) (Figure 3)

Then, we can eat an abundance of beans, lentils and chickpeas in our diet. They are our main protein source and so we eat them at least once every day—usually a spinach salad for lunch with beans on top. You can put loads of vegetables and beans in the salad and feel full without adding croutons or French dressing (which is processed). Instead, make a hummus-based dressing or use balsamic vinegar to flavor the salad. We find that the beans themselves are quite flavorful and often carry the taste of the salad.

> **CONSIDER ❸**
>
> √ **If you eat low calorie dense foods, you don't have to restrict your portions. You can take in the same amount of food and maybe even more but with that, you will take in fewer calories and still feel full.**

Oatmeal also is good for you, but adding bananas and raspberries makes it even better because it lowers the caloric density while adding the multiple benefits of the fruits. Eating bread is okay but adding hummus and an abundance of raw green vegetables makes it delicious and the vegetables lower the caloric density. A diet with these qualities is filling, and provides the essential nutrients required in daily living without the unnecessary toxins. Adding those raw veggies and fruits will make all the difference in reaching your wellness goals.

Our intention is not to restrict your portions. If you eat the right foods all of the time, you won't have to weigh yourself every day, or count points or calories. Throw away all of that nonsense! We want you to think about eating whole grains, and plant-based proteins such as legumes. We try to teach our patients how much of our lifestyle is correctable with diet. Learning to eat foods we aren't used to, or may not like, is difficult. We often tell our children that they don't have to like everything they eat, they just have to eat it. Our hope is that once they have tried eating enough healthier foods, they too will learn to love them.

Change is hard work. Eating healthy and exercising is hard work. For some, it will initially seem like an impossible task. People find it inconceivable to drink water in the morning with oatmeal and fruit, instead of coffee with cream and sugar and two pieces of buttered toast or processed cereals. People say to us that they don't care to change. They want to eat their meat and take their cholesterol medications too. Does that work? Unfortunately, it doesn't. Our cholesterol numbers might be better but our bodies are still inflamed, overweight and overtired. The body is still on fire. It all has to change.

With that in mind, you do the best you can. We drink caffeine. We just drink caffeinated teas without dairy. We break down occasionally and snack, but we often feel tired and uncomfortable when we do. We don't exercise every day. We don't sleep as much as we would like. Life happens. You do the best you can but every bit of change helps. You will find, though, that your energy is so much better with these changes. You won't have the highs and lows in energy based on the foods you eat because the food will be processed slowly in your system.

IS THIS A DIET?
THE PLANT-BASED LIFESTYLE

SO DOES THE PLANT-BASED LIFESTYLE WORK? ABSOLUTELY. In Dean Ornish's early work, he showed that with lifestyle modification, we can reverse heart disease. In his original work published in 1996, he directed 48 patients with moderate-severe coronary artery disease to make lifestyle changes. They were put on a 10-percent-fat vegetarian diet, encouraged to do moderate aerobic exercise, and were given stress management training and smoking cessation counseling. Over one year and more impressively over five years, plaque regression was noted in the treatment group and progression of

> **CONSIDER** ❹
> √ Think about the power of having a tool that acts like a medication without being one. These lifestyle changes not only stabilize plaque but may have the power to cause plaque regression.

atherosclerotic disease was noted in the control group.[155] The lifestyle changes worked! *(Consider 4)*

In 1995, an assessment of the Mediterranean diet, featuring an abundance of vegetables, fruit, and fiber, suggested that following the diet reduces heart disease risk. Further, researchers suggested that dairy intake is related to higher heart disease risk. Researchers in this trial also stated that the connection between higher dairy intake and lowering fracture rate is limited.[156] In another trial from 2002, it was noted that the optimal diet for lowering risk of coronary artery disease was a diet with non-hydrogenated fats, whole grains, and an abundance of fruits and vegetables.[157]

Many trials have examined the relationships between vegetables/ fruit and heart disease, and have shown an inverse relationship between increased consumption of fruits and vegetables and decreased risk of heart disease. The Lyons Diet study showed that eating more fruits and vegetables, and the alpha linoleic acid (ALA) found in the Mediterranean diet, reduced the incidence of myocardial infarctions (heart attacks) and mortality, compared with a regular low-fat diet.[158] Many more trials show the role of fruits and vegetables in lowering blood pressure.[159]

Regarding whole grains, the Iowa Women's Health Study showed that when people ate more whole grains, they suffered fewer cardiovascular events.[160] In the Nurses' Health Study, a 25-percent decrease in cardiovascular events was noted in women who ate more than three servings of whole grains per day versus those who ate less than one serving per day![161]

Two important studies highlight the benefits of a plant-based diet compared to the standard Western diet. In the Nurses' Health Study,[162] nurses were given either a whole-grain, plant-based diet versus the standard western diet, which is abundant in meat and processed meats, French fries and sweets. There was a 25-percent risk reduction in the whole-grain, plant-based diet compared to the standard Western diet. Similar results were also noted in the Health Professionals Follow-Up Study.[163]

There were also non-cardiovascular benefits to the Mediterranean diet. In the Nurses' Health Study, women who adopted this diet were found to have longer telomeres which, if you recall, are associated with longevity![164]

This data is compelling. It works. The data shows that the plant-based lifestyle is a healthier option than the alternative.

A WORD ON FERMENTED FOODS

FERMENTATION IS THE PROCESS of converting sugars to acids, gases or alcohol. It occurs in bacteria and yeast, and in our muscles when they are oxygen-depleted and lactic acid builds up. Fermentation creates many useful bacteria and enhances their nutritional effects with increased numbers of vitamins and omega-3 fatty acids. We view fermented foods as opportunities to naturally nourish our gut. They are natural probiotics. Examples of these fermented foods are kimchi (pickled vegetables from Korea), sauerkraut (fermented cabbage), kombucha (fermented mushrooms), miso (fermented soy) and tempeh (fermented soybeans). These are fabulous foods that we try to put into our diet a few times per week. You don't have to make them yourself; we buy jars of sauerkraut and kimchi and eat them with pita bread and hummus. We drink kombucha teas, cook with tempeh and eat miso soup. All good options to add the natural bacteria back into our bodies!

SO WHY NOT GO ON A DIET? BECAUSE THEY DON'T WORK

Research shows that approximately two-thirds of people who go on a specific weight-loss diet will fail to keep off the weight. A study published in American Psychologist reviewed 31 diet plans and their success rates; they found that after reaching their goal weights, one-third to two-thirds of the dieters regained not only the weight lost on the diet, but most gained even more weight than they had initially lost.[165] The authors of that study recognized that these percentages may be underestimating the actual incidence of weight regain, due to the way the follow-up programs were conducted. In eight of the studies, approximately 50 percent of the dieters did not participate in the follow-up surveys, and in many other studies the follow-up was done remotely (not in person), with no true measurements of weight by an independent party so people probably gained more weight than was recorded.

Most of us are not happy with failures in our lives, so many people may not have responded honestly to the remote survey as the pounds started creeping back on. But it may not be a personal failure that they failed to keep off the weight; people simply are not taught how to eat.

The key is to learn how to substitute whole, healthy foods that can then become your favorite foods. We hope to help you on this journey—not to give you a short-term "diet," but rather, to help you change your way of life.

For about the last 60 years in America, we've celebrated special occasions with sodas, sweet desserts, cakes, pies, candies and ice cream. As these foods have become readily available, many people have come to eat those high-calorie, nutrient-deficient foods every single day. But regularly consuming what used to be special-occasion highly caloric treats is making us overweight and obese. Many people drink sodas or other sweetened drinks all day long, every day of the week. Add that to fast food, donuts, other pastries and desserts, ice cream and other processed foods, and we are eating way too much processed sweeteners and flours, which are nutrient-poor, high-calorie foods.

Specific diets can be very difficult to maintain in the real world. Most diet plans do not address food addictions, dangers of processed sweeteners, necessity of fruits and vegetables, hydration, or a proper balance of complex carbohydrates, healthy proteins and fats. People are told to stop eating this and stop eating that, and not told what to eat instead. Many physicians say people cannot change and that we, as physicians, always recommend dietary changes, but most patients do not comply. People don't comply often because they haven't been taught how to eat. People need guidance and support. We think if people were presented the information in a positive way, we would see more people adopting healthier lifestyles.

There are also the diets that restrict one macronutrient: either protein, fats or carbohydrates. Many popular restrictive diets suggest restricting carbohydrates. You can lose a lot of weight quickly on a low-carbohydrate, high-protein, high-fat diet. Low-carb diets put the body into a state of ketosis, which is known to accelerate fat loss, which lures many people into trying it. For people who already enjoy eating high-protein, fatty foods such as bacon, steak, cheese and hamburgers, this sounds like the perfect answer. Eliminate or severely restrict carbohydrates and eat all the steak and bacon you can! Portion control is often not specified in these plans, so eating large portions may be encouraged. Some people may actually see elevated cholesterol levels on a high-fat, high-protein diet, even though they may be losing weight. *DO YOU KNOW HOW MANY STENTS WE HAVE PUT INTO PATIENTS WHO EAT LIKE THIS?*

Ketosis is the result of the body's burning fat for energy instead of burning the body's normal fuel, complex carbohydrates. People can actually test their urine to see if they are "in ketosis." Consuming large amounts of animal protein may be hard on the kidneys to begin with, and a prolonged state of ketosis might possibly stress the kidneys even more. This can be particularly difficult and potentially dangerous for those who are diabetic, pregnant or have been diagnosed with kidney disease.[166]

In these types of diets, the fact that the body needs the complex carbohydrates found in fresh fruits and vegetables is ignored. Complex carbohydrates normally provide fuel for the body and offer a huge variety of complex micronutrients and vitamins that can be lacking in most fats and proteins. Typically, once the weight loss has been achieved, the dieter will return to her previous eating habits with no knowledge of portion control or balanced nutrition. Again, weight gain most likely will occur.

Other diet plans suggest simply counting calories and/or counting carbohydrates. There are many new computer and smartphone apps that will track your consumption of calories and carbohydrates each day. These high-tech applications attempt to overcome the drudgery and complexity of all that counting. People don't understand that keeping track of only calories or carbohydrates does not show you the nutritional quality of those calories. Simply reducing calories is not the answer. People also feel hungry all of the time. Recall, legumes and beans cause butyrate production which triggers leptin and tells us we are full. Counting carbs and cutting calories make us feel hungry and unsatisfied. Ironically, counting is not necessary when one is consuming a whole-food diet of predominantly fresh vegetables, legumes (dried beans and lentils), fruits and whole grains.

BOTTOM LINE: Overeating, drinking sodas (sweetened or artificially sweetened), dehydration, eating predominantly packaged foods and lack of exercise are the major causes of most obesity in America today. Diets do not work; eating healthy, whole fresh foods, avoiding packaged foods, staying hydrated and exercising regularly are the formula for achieving and maintaining a healthy weight. It sounds difficult, but you can begin simply by making small changes—drink a glass of water in the morning, go for a walk, buy some fresh vegetables and fruits, read the labels on any packaged foods you may want to buy. This is your life—choose health!

Many people think it is too expensive to eat healthy whole foods, but it really isn't, it just takes a little bit of planning. Brown rice, lentils, quinoa and dried beans are some of the least expensive foods available. They offer plenty of nutrients, fiber, vitamins and minerals. Cooked dry beans are another excellent source of fiber and protein. Shopping for fresh local vegetables and fruits at local farmer's markets and buying frozen vegetables and fruits at the grocery store are other effective ways to minimize your costs for healthy food options. Remember to always read the labels on packaged foods to ensure there have been no added sweeteners or other unhealthy ingredients. Be sure the only ingredient is the actual fruit or vegetable. ▪

YOUR PRESCRIPTION:
Eat Smart

The right food choices can make a big diffence in your health

❶ **Try to get in 5-7 servings of fruits and vegetables** per day. Eat more vegetables than fruit.

❷ **Eat lots of colorful vegetables** every day.

❸ **Learn to eat beans and lentils** every day.

❹ **Don't be afraid of the carb.** Eat whole grains. You will feel great and weight loss will be a side effect.

CHAPTER 9:

Oil Change: Nuts, Seeds And Avocado

What is the deal with fats and oils?

FAT CONSUMPTION is necessary for our development, so it's important to discuss. Fats can be broken down into saturated fats and unsaturated fats. Unsaturated fats are further broken down into monounsaturated fats (MUFAs) and polyunsaturated fats (PUFAs). PUFAs are further broken down into the essential fatty acids (EFAs): omega-3 and omega-6 fatty acids. Let's go through this in more detail now. *(Figure 1)*

SATURATED FATS:

SATURATED FATS ARE SOLID AT ROOM TEMPERATURE. They are very stable and have a long shelf life. The most common saturated fats are butter and animal fats such as milk, cheese and meat. Plant substances that are saturated fats are coconut oil, palm oil, palm kernel oil and cocoa butter. The general feeling is that saturated fats should be avoided because they will increase risk of cardiovascular disease. In 1908, rabbits were given a high cholesterol/high saturated fat diet and their atherosclerosis (hardening of the arteries) increased.[167] In the 1950s, studies showed that a diet rich in saturated fats and cholesterol was associated with higher cholesterol levels in humans.[168] Epidemiologic studies performed around that time also showed that higher cholesterol predicted one's risk of coronary heart disease.[169] This led to the diet-heart hypothesis which postulated that eating saturated fats and cholesterol can lead to heart disease.[170]

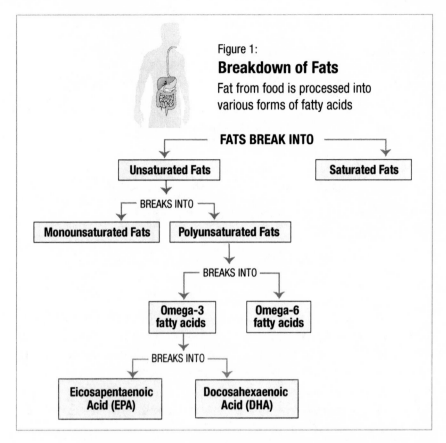

Figure 1:
Breakdown of Fats
Fat from food is processed into various forms of fatty acids

FATS BREAK INTO

Unsaturated Fats

Saturated Fats

BREAKS INTO

Monounsaturated Fats

Polyunsaturated Fats

BREAKS INTO

Omega-3 fatty acids

Omega-6 fatty acids

BREAKS INTO

Eicosapentaenoic Acid (EPA)

Docosahexaenoic Acid (DHA)

Support for this hypothesis significantly increased after the seven countries study[171] in the 1970s which strongly associated saturated fats with coronary heart disease. Since that time, saturated fats have been considered the unhealthy fat.

Saturated fats are very useful for the food industry, however, because they have a long shelf life. Foods made with lard and other animal fats last longer. When saturated fats were thought to be unhealthy, food producers had to reconsider how foods were being prepared. Interest shifted to unsaturated fats.

THE SHIFT TO POLYUNSATURATED FATS:

WHEN SATURATED FATS FELL OUT OF VOGUE, food producers started looking at unsaturated fats as an alternative. We mentioned that unsaturated fats are broken into PUFAs and MUFAs. PUFAs are fats that are liquid at room temperature, such as vegetable oils (corn oil), but they also can be found in sources such as whole grains, nuts and seeds. When we extract the oils from corn (corn oil), seeds and other vegetables, we are extracting pure fat. All of the beneficial fiber is removed as well as many of the other nutrients found in the whole food itself. Most processed oils are used in packaged foods/processed foods and for cooking, in salad dressings and dips. PUFAs are thought to be beneficial because they're comprised of omega-3 and omega-6 fatty acids as discussed below.

OMEGA-3 FATTY ACIDS

OMEGA-3 FATTY ACIDS HAVE BEEN STUDIED extensively, mostly from marine sources. Studies suggest that omega-3 fatty acids may lower your risk of abnormal heart rhythms.[172] They help to reduce triglycerides (fat in the blood), aid in blood thinning and may help to improve dilatation of blood vessels.[173] Fish has been shown in people who consume two or more servings per week to increase lifespan.[174] In studies, these improvements in lifespan were noted with marine omega-3 fatty acids and were most notable when intake was as high as 30 percent of the overall intake. Omega-3 fatty acids are comprised of eicosapentaenoic acid (EPA) and docosahexaenoic acid (DHA) which have been shown to be key factors in decreasing coronary heart disease.[175] Alpha-linoleic acid (ALA) is an omega-3 fatty acid found in plant sources such as flaxseed, canola oil and soybean oil and can be converted to EPA and DHA in the body. ALA has been shown to improve cardiovascular outcomes and decrease heart disease.[176,177] *(Figure 2)*

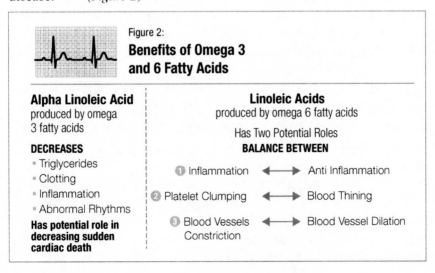

Figure 2:
Benefits of Omega 3 and 6 Fatty Acids

Alpha Linoleic Acid
produced by omega 3 fatty acids

DECREASES
* Triglycerides
* Clotting
* Inflammation
* Abnormal Rhythms

Has potential role in decreasing sudden cardiac death

Linoleic Acids
produced by omega 6 fatty acids

Has Two Potential Roles
BALANCE BETWEEN

1. Inflammation ←→ Anti Inflammation
2. Platelet Clumping ←→ Blood Thining
3. Blood Vessels Constriction ←→ Blood Vessel Dilation

OMEGA-6 FATTY ACIDS:

BESIDES OMEGA-3 FATTY ACIDS, there is much discussion about omega-6 fatty acids. You'll recall that unsaturated fats can be divided into omega-3 and omega-6 fatty acids. Many people feel that omega-3 fatty acids are the "good" fatty acids and omega-6 fatty acids are the "bad" ones. However, is that really true? The main omega-6 fatty acid is linoleic acid (different from alpha-linoleic acid made by omega-3 fatty acids). Linoleic acid is found in foods such as corn, soy, sunflower and safflower. When linoleic acid is ingested, it breaks down into eicosanoids, some of which promote inflammation and platelet aggregation (potential for plaque formation) and tightening of the blood vessels. However, some of the eicosanoids have the opposite effect and promote anti-inflammation, decrease platelet aggregation and dilate blood vessels. We are not entirely clear of the percentages of each eicosanoid that each food creates or what is the optimal balance in our bodies. *(Figure 2)*

We typically think of inflammation, platelet aggregation and tightening of the blood vessels as "bad" things, but the body certainly needs some omega-6 fats from the diet for proper blood clotting and appropriate inflammation to heal the body's injuries. If we didn't clot, we could bleed out when we cut ourselves or fall and skin a knee! Remember that inflammation is a normal response to a bodily insult. It is the body's response to stress. That stress triggers the body to heal and respond to the attack. However, with continuous stress on the body, the body becomes imbalanced and that triggers uncontrolled inflammation. Then, it can be seen that we need some amounts of both omega-3 and omega-6 fatty acids. The right balance, however is not so clear.

Why don't we know what is the right balance of omega-3 and omega-6 acids? The problem is that human trials of omega-6 fatty acids are imperfect. We have some data showing that higher doses of omega-6 fatty acids can cause oxidation (not good) of LDL and may promote inflammation.[178] Other studies suggest that all PUFAs (omega-3 and omega-6 fatty acids both) are associated with narrowing of blood vessels.[179] In contrast, some studies suggest an LDL-lowering effect of omega-6 fatty acids when omega-6 PUFAs were substituted for saturated fats.[180] This, however, may not be because omega-6 PUFAs are good in isolation but that they are better than saturated fats.

Unfortunately, there are no clinical trials that specifically look at outcomes from adding omega-6 fatty acids to the diet and assessing outcomes. Many observational studies show either a small benefit from additional omega-6 fatty acids or no benefit at all.[181] However, two studies show that the omega-6 fatty acid, linoleic acid, was associated with decreased heart disease.[182] Overall, the American Heart Association now suggests that 5-10 percent of our diets should be omega-6 fatty acids, which may bring about a decrease in coronary heart disease. [183]

How much omega-6 fatty acid we should include in our diets, and what ratio of omega-3 to omega-6, continues to be debated. Likely, we should attain a balance in our diets between the two. Currently, however, the average American diet has 14 to 25 times more omega-6 than omega-3.[184] The Mediterranean diet appears to have much a better balance of omega-3 to omega-6 and is closer to what we think people should follow. All types of fatty acids appear to have a beneficial role to some degree, but we are likely getting too much omega-6 fatty acid in our diet. It is suggested that a 1:1 or 1:2 balance of omega-6 to omega-3 fats would provide the proper balance for optimal health, allowing the body to clot and heal when injured, but also controlling inflammation and clotting when we are not injured.

So what does that mean in terms of the foods we should eat? *(Figure 3, page 112)* When we look at oils, the ratio of omega-6 to omega-3 fatty acids is highest in corn oil (48:1), followed by sunflower oil (13:1), then olive oil (13:1). (Important: olive oil is 72 percent monounsaturated fat and the remainder is polyunsaturated fat). Vegetable and soybean oils then follow at 9:1 and 8:1 respectively. (courtesy of Jeff Novick, RD). Canola oil (rapeseed oil) has a ratio of about 2:1. Flaxseed oil is probably the healthiest oil, with little

√ CONSIDER 1

Flax seed oil is a great oil in terms of best ratio of omega 3:6 fatty acids but you can't cook with it because heating it makes it potentially harmful to the body.

* You can add it to a smoothie.

* You can also add flax seeds to foods after they have been cooked.

* You can add ground flax seeds into your oatmeal after it is cooked. Or add them to a cereal or smoothie

* Seeds should be ground otherwise, the seeds will often pass through the body unprocessed and we don't yield the benefits.

* It is okay to bake with flax seed meal (think about with bread, cakes, muffins).

Figure 3:

SOURCES OF HIGH CONCENTRATIONS
OF OMEGA-3 FATTY ACIDS:

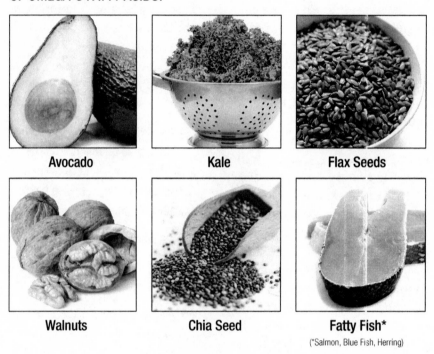

Avocado	Kale	Flax Seeds
Walnuts	Chia Seed	Fatty Fish*

(*Salmon, Blue Fish, Herring)

saturated fat, a large proportion of polyunsaturated fat and a good ratio of omega-6 to omega-3 fatty acids. Of note, however, flaxseed cannot be used to cook with because it is potentially harmful when warmed. *(Consider 1)*

THE TRANS-FATS

HISTORICALLY SPEAKING, the benefits of PUFAs in decreasing heart disease were compelling and well touted but the food industry struggled because of their poor shelf life. As a result, manufacturers began hydrogenating the oils to make them easier to use and longer-lasting. This began the advent of the trans-fat years. It was easy for manufacturers to use trans-fats because they were not saturated fats, which had become unpopular due to their potential cardiovascular effects; what's more, trans-fats were polyunsaturated fats so they were considered healthy and when they were hydrogenated, they had the added benefit of a longer shelf life. Without realizing it, however, the manufacturers added highly toxic oils back into our systems that actually are more toxic to our hearts than saturated fats.

Controlled studies have shown that trans-fats increase LDL and lower HDL cholesterol, compared to non-hydrogenated unsaturated fatty acids.[185] They also increase lipoprotein[a] (a pro-inflammatory marker)[186], increase triglycerides [187] and may reduce the blood vessel's ability to dilate. Trans-fats also increase our risk of diabetes.[188] Over the years, the clinical trials have become better; they're larger and more randomized and show the negative impact of trans-fats on the risk of coronary heart disease.[189] The Nurses' Health Study looked at 80,082 women and found that higher trans-fats (and, to a smaller extent, saturated fats) were associated with higher risk of heart disease compared to the polyunsaturated non-hydrogenated diet.[190]

During the trans-fat years, people started looking at the Mediterranean diet more closely. Studies began showing that the Mediterranean diet was linked to a lower cardiovascular mortality. Analysis of food oils used in this diet led to the focus on olive oil as the "golden oil" and targeted the abundance of MUFAs and PUFAs in the oil. Olive oil is 72 percent monounsaturated fat. The remainder is linoleic acid which, as you may recall, is an omega-6 polyunsaturated fat. MUFAs have been shown to lower triglycerides and LDL levels and elevate HDL compared to saturated fats. In some studies, they have been shown to improve cardiovascular outcomes,[191] ease oxidative stress and improve diabetes control. Olive oil is also rich in polyphenols which are believed to decrease oxidative stresses on the cells (reduce cell damage).[192]

To date, olive oil has enjoyed the spotlight as the oil used in the Mediterranean diet and therefore, has been purported as the oil that can improve heart health. People often will add olive oil to their foods because of its cardiovascular benefits, above and beyond their normal food requirements. Many of our patients explain that they are eating olive oil because it is good for the heart. But is that the right thing to do? The BIG QUESTION: Is olive oil or any oil actually good for us by itself? Or is it just better than the alternatives—saturated and trans-fats?

A study in 1995 was performed on African green monkeys.[193] They were fed three different diets: one high in monounsaturated fats, one high in polyunsaturated fats and one high in saturated fats. LDL cholesterol ("lousy" cholesterol-we want this low) was fairly similar in the mono-and poly-unsaturated groups, which was lower than the saturated fat group. The HDL cholesterol (good cholesterol-we want this high) was similar between the saturated fat and the monounsaturated fats and lowest in the polyunsaturated fats. When you look at coronary artery disease in these monkeys, though, regardless of the type of fat in their diet, they all developed atherosclerosis—clogging of the arteries. The amount of disease was similar between the monounsaturated and saturated fat groups. So if all groups despite the food being primarily full of mono-, poly- or saturated fats developed heart disease, is oil ever really a good thing?

Interestingly, atherosclerotic plaque was lowest in the polyunsaturated group, which actually had the lowest levels of that good HDL cholesterol. This was likely due to changes in LDL particle composition and higher amount of omega-3 fatty acids. Jeff Novick, when he was at the Pritikin Center,[194] also noted a University of Crete study. In that study, researchers looked retrospectively at patients with heart disease and those who were heart-healthy, and found that those who had heart disease had a diet higher in olive oil and fats compared to those who did not. It was more information supporting the notion that oil of any type causes heart plaque.

> ## √ CONSIDER 2
>
> Olive oil is NOT the "wonder" oil. There is no oil that is good for us. Having no oil is better than any of the oils. All oils have the ability to cause heart plaque.

More information was found when looking at the work of Dr. A's former mentors, Dr. Robert Vogel and colleagues at the University of Maryland. Drs. Vogel, Coretti and Plotnick did a study[195] in which they looked at dilatation of blood vessels by giving subjects food that emphasized different portions of the Mediterranean diet (olive oil, canola oil and salmon). They found that patients who received canola oil or salmon actually had the ability to open their blood vessels compared to the other groups. On the other, olive oil caused a reduction in the size of the blood vessels. In their conclusion, they noted that a diet full of antioxidant-rich foods such as fruits, vegetables, fish, vinegar and canola oils are the important parts of the Mediterranean diet, rather than the olive oil. Here again, the findings point out that perhaps olive oil is not the wonder oil that it has been purported to be. (Consider 2)

All three classes of fatty acids (saturated fats, monounsaturated fats and polyunsaturated fats) increase HDL when they replace carbohydrates in the diet. This increase is slightly higher in monounsaturated fats than with saturated fats. Monounsaturated fats are believed to lower cholesterol more than saturated fats when replacing saturated fats on a pound-per-pound basis. As such, it is not that these oils were thought to be healthy; they were just seen as better than the saturated fats they were replacing.

When the components of the Mediterranean diet were carefully analyzed, a few important points were realized: *(Consider 3)*

1. **Consumption of fruits, vegetables and legumes** decreased mortality; i.e., the more you eat, the less likely you are to die.

2. **That mortality ratio was equal for fish and seafood**, meaning there is no mortality benefit or detriment from eating fish.

3. **With respect to dairy and meat**, a positive association was found between consumption and mortality; so the more consumption, the higher the mortality risk.[196]

CALORIE DENSITY OF OILS

CALORIC DENSITY REFERS TO the calories per gram or pound of a substance. Olive oil, pound per pound, is one of the most caloric-dense substances and the most calorie-dense oil. One tablespoon of olive oil typically provides 14 grams of fat (just over 120 calories, all from fat)! Oil makes us gain weight with a slight increase in HDL and still causes plaque in the heart.

√ **CONSIDER 3**

When the components of the Mediterranean diet were analyzed three main points were derived.

❶ **Consumption of fruits, vegetables and legumes decreased mortality;** i.e., there more you eat, the less likely you are to die.

❷ **That mortality ratio was equal** for fish and seafood, meaning there was no mortality benefit or detriment from eating fish.

❸ **With respect to dairy and meat,** there was a positive association between consumption and mortality; so the more consumption, the larger the mortality risk.

Now, let's get back to the question of whether saturated fats are so bad? Do we know for sure that saturated fats are bad and unsaturated fats are good? Yes and no. Many meta-analyses show that a higher dietary intake of cholesterol and saturated fats increases cholesterol in the blood, and we further know that high cholesterol is associated with increased mortality.[197] A recent meta-anaylsis published in 2014[198] states that saturated fats are not associated with increased cardiovascular risk, and the only beneficial fats are PUFAs when they replaced saturated fats because of their higher levels of omega-3 fatty acids. This trial came under great criticism because of its observational nature with multiple confounding affects. Therefore, the American Heart Association still believes that we should eat a diet low in saturated fats and high in whole grains, fruits and vegetables. We still believe that vegetable oils are better than animal fats, but just by a bit. They all cause plaque in the heart and make us gain weight. So it is not that any oil is good for us but rather, that some oils are somewhat less bad than other options.

AVOCADO

LET'S TALK ABOUT THE AVOCADO for a moment because it has come under a great deal of scrutiny. Avocados are highly potent fruits. They are full of potassium, magnesium, iron, B vitamins, and vitamins C and E. They possess the carotenoid, lutein which is good for our eyes and folate which is crucial for cell repair. Avocados are high in fat, though, so they are calorie-dense fruits. Overall, they are rich in omega-3 fatty acids (good) and MUFAs. Remember, we have learned that all of these fats can still cause plaque in the heart. However, does the benefit of the avocado outweigh the negative of the fat? For patients with known heart disease or multiple risk factors, avocado may have to be restricted. However, for many, the avocado is a filling, nutrient-rich option to add a plant based, whole grain diet.

A WORD ON COCONUT OIL

TO FINISH THE HISTORICAL ASSESSMENT OF OIL, we need to talk about coconut and palm oils. After trans-fats were banned, the food industry started looking again for other oils that were not animal-based and had a long shelf life. The search for "good fats" was becoming something of a journey: first, saturated fats were used in abundance. Then, negative effects were discovered. PUFAs were felt to be good but had poor shelf life. We found later that hydrogenating the PUFAs to make trans-fats was actually worse. People shifted to non-hydrogenated PUFAs and MUFAs.

The food industry started asking if there were any other options? They continued to look for cheap, palatable oils with long shelf life. This brought the conversation to coconut and palm kernel oil. Unfortunately, we have very little trial data on these oils and their benefits.

Palm kernel oil and coconut oil are primarily saturated fats. Coconut oil is made of 90 percent saturated fats. The remainder is a small amount of unsaturated fat, primarily omega-6 fatty acids.

What do we know about coconut oil? Not much, really. We know from early studies that saturated fats increase our risk of cardiovascular mortality and that the hydrogenated forms of coconut oils that were popular in the 1980s were extremely harmful. We learned from the monkey studies that all oils cause atherosclerotic disease. Coconut oil also doesn't have a good omega 3:6 ratio so it appears to be pro-inflammatory. Is there more to it, though? Why has it become popular?

Coconut oil is different from other saturated fats because it is primarily made of medium-chain triglycerides (lauric acid). There is some preliminary data on its role in preventing Alzheimer's disease. One trial from 2009[199] looked at 20 women aged 20 to 40 years. They were asked to eat a low-calorie diet and walk 50 minutes every day. They were given 30 mL of soybean oil or coconut oil. The coconut oil group was noted to have slightly higher HDL (49 gm/dL versus 45 gm/dL) and a slightly better LDL/HDL ratio. This difference was quite small, though. There was also an association regarding weight loss in the coconut oil group.

Because coconut oil is made of medium-chain fatty acids instead of long-chain fatty acids like most other fats, some scientists believe it is not stored as fat deposits. It may even be associated with fat burning. It may allow for more efficient processing of fat. Data from studies performed on mice show that those who were given medium-chain fatty acids had less muscle fatigue. So does coconut oil deserve the hype it has received? Unfortunately, very little is known about this oil and we would suggest it be used with caution. An oil that is 90 percent saturated fats concerns us. We know that in the African monkeys studies, plaque formed in all the monkeys' vessels regardless of the type of oil they were given.

WHAT ABOUT NUTS AND SEEDS?

NUTS AND SEEDS HAVE BECOME VERY POPULAR lately as heart-healthy foods. Nuts and seeds are packed with unsaturated fats, both mono and polyunsaturated fats. Then, because they have PUFAs, they also are rich in omega-3 and omega-6 fatty acids. Nuts also have fiber which helps lower our cholesterol and makes us feel full. They also contain vitamin E, which may play a role in reducing heart plaque development. Importantly, nuts have plant sterols which help to lower cholesterol. They are known to also decrease oxidative stress[200] and they are rich in L-arginine which may help with dilatation of the blood vessels and make them less prone to clogs.[201] *(Figure 3) (Consider 4)*

It is important to remember that nuts are high in caloric density so they should not be eaten in great numbers, and not regularly. While nuts were again part of the Mediterranean diet, they were not a large enough portion of the diet to justify high intakes.

> ## √ CONSIDER 4
>
> Nuts are filled with unsaturated fats. They have fiber and plant sterols which lower cholesterol, decrease oxidative stress and dilate our blood vessels. Overall, nuts are a good part of our diets, in moderation.

There is a lot of interesting data on nuts. The Adventist Health Study[202] is one that showed people who ate nuts more than four times per week had fewer cardiovascular events compared to those who consumed less than one serving per week. Serving size was about one ounce, two to five times per week. In another study, when a small group of men following a restricted diet and fairly equivalent fats and calories shifted 20 percent of their fats/calories to come from walnuts, their total cholesterol dropped, as well as both their LDL and HDL cholesterols.[203] In the Nurses' Health Study,[204] there also appeared to be a beneficial effect to eating nuts in terms of decreasing heart disease. But, this is observational data and while the nurses who ate nuts had less heart disease, those nurses also exercised more, ate less meat, were leaner and smoked less. *(Consider 5)*

A meta-analysis from 2010 examined trials that involved giving people who ate diets with equal amounts of saturated fats, either nuts or no nuts. It was the first time that we clearly saw a benefit from eating nuts. The difference was noted as a drop in total cholesterol (5 percent) and the reduction in LDL cholesterol (7 percent).[205] The study also noted that the response was dose-related; i.e. the more nuts, the more significant the impact (1.3 ounces versus 2.4 to 2.6 ounces). Importantly, the study also showed that the greatest impact was seen in people who replaced their saturated fats with nuts rather than using nuts to replace olive oil or carbohydrates. So, this shows us that if we continue to eat the Western diet full of

> ## √ CONSIDER 5
>
> Goal serving size of nuts: 1 oz of nuts 2-5 times per week

saturated fats, exchanging them for nuts is of benefit. In people who already have a low saturated fat diet, the impact is less.

What is the best nut? Walnuts are known to be high in fiber, rich in antioxidants and full of alpha-linoleic acid, a plant based omega-3 fatty acid. There are studies on walnuts that show improvement in the dilation of blood vessels when given to men in exchange for one-third of their monounsaturated fats.[206]

Peanuts, which are actually legumes, are rich in monounsaturated fat, magnesium and folate. Studies show that dietary fiber, arginine and magnesium increased in the peanut eating group, which may improve cardiovascular outcomes.[207]

Cashews are abundant in magnesium. Brazil nuts contain selenium, which may help to protect against prostate cancer, and deficiencies in selenium can cause weakening of the heart. Almonds are rich in fiber, vitamin E and monounsaturated fats. They have been also shown to decrease LDL by small numbers and improve other cardiovascular parameters.[208]

There also is data to show that pecans, hazelnuts, macadamia nuts and pistachios all have lipid lowering abilities. But which one should you eat? Truthfully, we have read all the trials. There is data on many of the nuts. If we had to choose one nut that was better than the rest, we would probably pick the walnut. But other

> √ **CONSIDER 6**
>
> What is the best nut? Probably, the walnut but all nuts have some benefits.

than that, we also think that all nuts have some benefit. *(Consider 6)*

So the bottom line is that nuts are a good addition to our diets. They are best when they are used instead of oils, dairy and meats. They are a great addition to a whole-food, plant-based diet. We should eat about a handful, three to five times per week, and that is likely adequate. They are calorie dense and eating too many will cause weight gain.

WHAT ABOUT SEEDS?

Seeds are plant foods that are rich in protein. Again, few studies have been done on seeds, so unfortunately, we have little data at this point. Chia seeds and flaxseeds are probably the best seeds you can eat. Chia seeds date back to 3500 BC during the time of the Aztecs, who ate them regularly, and are abundant in fiber, calcium and manganese. They also are the seed with the most alpha-linoleic acid (ALA), which you may recall has benefits for the heart, perhaps as a precursor for omega-3 fatty acids. In the Lyon Heart Study that looked at the Mediterranean diet, the diet was rich in ALA, which significantly lowered heart disease risk.[209],[210] Importantly, in that study, the benefits from the ALA were found apart from the benefits from the fish (marine source of omega-3 fatty acids), suggesting that the benefits from the ALA were additive.

How to eat chia seeds? Small studies show that grinding chia seeds boosts the levels of omega-3 fatty acids in our blood. They also have been associated with higher energy and a feeling of fullness. Eating a teaspoon, ground, a few times per week is probably adequate. *(Consider 7)*

> ## √ CONSIDER 7
>
> How to eat chia seeds? Grind you seeds to increase to increase the absorption of omega-3 fatty acids in blood. Have 1 tsp of ground chia seeds a few times per week

Similar to chia seeds, flaxseeds have also been around for centuries. They bring many benefits because they are also rich in alpha-linoleic acid and contain lignans, which are plant estrogens and may play a role in reducing the risk of breast cancer, at least in laboratory animals. Lignans appear to be anti-inflammatory as well, and have been shown in small studies to lower cholesterol levels. Flaxseeds keep best when whole, but they should be ground before eating them to get their maximum potency. One teaspoon ground is likely adequate a couple of times per week.

Before we continue, we want to caution readers on portion sizes and how often we should eat nuts and seeds. We do not feel a person should be eating one teaspoon of chia, walnuts, or flaxseed every day. All foods should be varied. We are giving general parameters. Do not eat all of these things every day because you don't need that much and people are often frustrated with weight gain. VARY IT UP!

What about other seeds? Pumpkin seeds are high in protein and fiber. They also are rich in L-tryptophan, which can help with moods and depression. They are also rich in most B-complex vitamins (not B12, however). Pomegranate seeds are also important seeds. Pomegranate has been shown in studies to decrease plaque formation in blood vessels (thus reducing heart disease). Sesame seeds are also high in fiber and calcium, and are full of lignans, similar to flax seeds. Sunflower seeds are rich in vitamin E and plant sterols, which appear to lower cholesterol. Cumin seeds, which have been around for centuries have antiseptic properties. *(Consider 8)*

People often want to know how much to take and how often. At the end of the day, there is no cocktail recipe. These nuts and seeds should be part of a whole-grain, plant-based diet. They should be remembered for their calcium, B vitamins and fiber. They should be remembered as rich in alpha-linoleic acid and lignans.

A BRIEF NOTE ON CHILDREN

WHILE CAUTION needs to be used with adults, we believe there is more room for flexibility with children. While we prefer they don't eat oils and animal products, they do need more caloric density that their adult counterparts. So don't hold back on nuts, seeds and avocado with your children, and do let them have a little oil. Just use the oil in moderation for children and make up the caloric density with nuts and seeds.

People often ask Dr. A if she raises her children exclusively on a whole-grain, plant-based diet. Dr A: "The answer is that at home, I cook exclusively plant-based. I feed them lots of lentils, beans and greens. Initially, I would tell them they had to eat the food that I prepared because it was healthy. Now, they love the foods. It takes 10 times to love something. Now my kids ask for spinach, hummus and lentils. But if the kids go to a birthday party and eat macaroni and cheese or chicken or we go out to dinner, I don't stop them. I am not running a dictatorship and a diet that they will later rebel against. Kids need to figure it out themselves. We offer them a healthy lifestyle at home and I hope that with time, they will realize the difference in how they feel when they eat the foods that are good for them. Truthfully, with a few exceptions, my kids love to eat plant-based!"

> ## √ CONSIDER 8
>
> People often don't think about adding seeds to their diets. Remember them when making a salad to bulk the salad up. Add to breads, cereals and cold soups. They can be added to smoothies too!

A healthy diet is not about any one food item. It is not about eating three grams of fish oil or flaxseeds. It is not only about kale or limiting yourself to eating just walnuts or vegetables. It is also not about eating high-fat, processed foods and then adding nuts or kale and expect to make it all better. It is about the whole thing. When people try to tease out what is great about the Mediterranean diet, or any diet for that matter, they often are looking for that one magic food that is going to heal us. We have to put work into this lifestyle and learn how to complement foods so we get a balanced diet. Magic foods don't exist. There is no one ingredient that makes our health better. It is the whole thing—a balance. Once we understand that, then the true healing can begin. *

YOUR PRESCRIPTION:

Finding Your Good Food Balance

❶ Try to decrease oil intake in general. No oil is really good for you. Try to be creative by using water or orange juice to sauté.

❷ If you want to add oil for taste, the best oil is probably flaxseed oil. However, you cannot heat flaxseed oil because it makes the good fats unhealthy. It's best to use flaxseeds in baking or add them to morning cereal, shakes or oatmeal. Consider eating them in a salad.

❸ Canola and olive oils are probably the best oils to cook with. But remember, there are no wonder oils.

❹ If you feel as if you need more substance, eat nuts, seeds and avocado. They are calorie-dense and will make you feel full, but too many will cause weight gain.

❺ There is no magic food. There is no food you can eat that will balance out the bad foods you're eating. Eat balanced. Be creative and learn how to make fabulous food that is tasty and great for you.

CHAPTER 10:

Spice It Up With The Spices (and Herbs) of Life

The flavorful and ancient anti-inflammatory medicine cabinet in our kitchens

SPICES ARE AN ESSENTIAL PART of a whole-grain, plant-based diet. They are very potent in decreasing inflammation and have many medicinal properties. Spices have been an important part of life for millennia, long praised for their flavors, smells and medicinal properties. There are Egyptian documents tracing the use of spices as early as 1500-2000 BCE where the role of spices as medicine was appreciated. These documents note the benefits of anise, mustard, saffron and cinnamon. Notably, cinnamon is not endemic to ancient Egypt, suggesting spice trading occurred that long ago. Egyptians used cinnamon for mummification. Cinnamon was put in vials and placed in pharaohs' coffins to accompany them to the afterlife.

Notes written in 950 BCE mention an incense route followed by traders carrying spices from Asia to Europe. Spices were coveted and traded for large sums of gold and silver. When Alexander the Great conquered Egypt in 80 BCE, he established Alexandria as a port for spice trade. Romans and Greeks viewed spices as markers of wealth and luxury; they would heap it on banquet tables and use it in making spice-scented perfumes. They valued spices' medicinal properties. During the 8th to 15th centuries, spice trade was an important form of commerce dominated by the Republic of Venice. Spices were moved from Asia to Europe with the help of Arab middlemen.[211]

In the 15th century, Spain and Portugal attempted to thwart the Venetian monopoly and sent Christopher Columbus to find India via a western route. It was on that trip that he discovered America. Over the following centuries, the Dutch, Spanish, French and British colonized all the countries that could provide an abundance of spices. By the end of the 17th century, the Dutch East India Company was the richest corporation in the world, showing how much spices were valued.

Why are spices important for good health? They are concentrated forms of the most potent parts of the plants they come from. Spices are full of phytonutrients. Recall, phytonutrients are involved in cell signaling and communication; that is, the information pathway in the body. We have established that phytonutrients are found in our fruits and vegetables. However, some phytonutrients can be found only in spices. When phytonutrients are involved in cell signaling, they can help turn markers in the inflammatory cascade on and off. In that way, spices can be beneficial in reducing inflammation and oxidative stresses.

So what do spices contain that can be found nowhere else? Certain vital phytonutrients can only be garnered from spices. For instance, curcumin, a vital anti-inflammatory with anti-cancer benefits, can only be found in turmeric. Thymoquinone is a potent immune booster and only exists in black cumin. Piperine has neuroprotective effects (protects the brain cells) and is unique to black pepper. Eugenol, found only in cloves, is a powerful pain killer. Rosmarinic acid is a potent antioxidant and the only source is rosemary. Capsaicin is a great medication for arthritis and its only source is chili peppers. The list goes on and on. Spices provide a long list of benefits that can't be found anywhere else. *(Figure 1)*

When writing this book, we had to think hard about which spices we wanted to discuss because so many of them deliver fabulous health benefits. We decided to present some of our favorites—but first we want to mention an enlightening book by Dr. Bharat Aggarwal (no relation to authors) called *Healing Spices*,[212] in which he brilliantly outlines an abundance of spices and their benefits. Our all-time favorite spice is TURMERIC, often called "India's gold." We call this spice our gold, too.

TURMERIC: OUR GOLD

FOR CENTURIES, INDIANS have been studied because they suffer very little chronic illness. Yes, diseases of poverty and poor medical attention are rampant, but chronic illness is not—at least it wasn't until the modern era. This is likely because of the "thrift theory:" For

FIGURE 1:

CERTAIN PHYTONUTRIENTS can only be found in spices

	SPICES	ACTIVE INGREDIENTS	ACTION
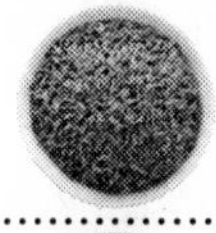	**Black Cumin**	Thymoquinone	Immune Booster
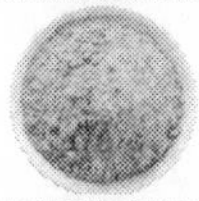	**Turmeric**	Curcumin	Anti-Inflammatory
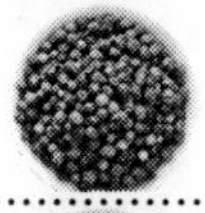	**Black Pepper**	Piperine	Protects Brain Cells
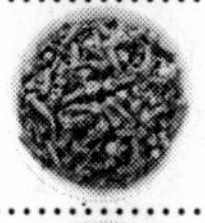	**Cloves**	Eugenol	Pain Killer
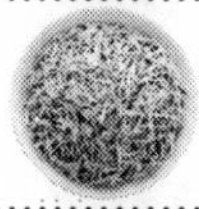	**Rosemary**	Rosmarinic Acid	Anti-Oxidant
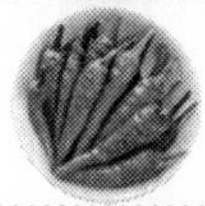	**Chili**	Capsaicin	Pain Reliever

centuries, Indian people lived in villages and walked as their form of transportation. They subsisted on diets consisting primarily of rice, vegetables, nuts and seeds—and an abundance of spices. Turmeric is one of those spices that is widespread in that country, and many believe it is the reason Indians have less chronic illness.

So why is turmeric so great? Turmeric's vital ingredient is curcumin. It provides a wide variety of benefits, and one of its most important merits is its anti-inflammatory quality. Turmeric has been shown to decrease inflammation in joints and reduce symptoms of arthritis. In a recent study, one group of patients took 2000mg of turmeric compared to participants who took 800mg of ibuprofen. Researchers found that

> ### √ CONSIDER 1
>
> Turmeric can be used to treat arthritis pain instead of ibuprofen

turmeric provided at least as much relief from patients' symptom as ibuprofen, and without the side effects that come from taking anti-inflammatory medications. Just think about that for a second![213] *(Consider 1)*

Turmeric is considered a powerful antioxidant. It has been shown in animal studies to lower our risk of cancers such as breast, colon, prostate, and even skin cancers when ingested regularly. The incidence of cancer in India is much lower than that of its Western counterparts. [214]

Turmeric may also play a role in treating Alzheimer's disease, due the spice's anti-inflammatory effects. Our brains contain cells called neurons that are responsible for connecting so that our thoughts can manifest in actions. But in people with Alzheimer's disease, plaque forms between these cells, reducing the ability of these neurons to communicate. These communications are the key to cognition, memory and judgment and without these functions we see the impairments evident in Alzheimer's patients. Triggers for Alzheimer's disease are likely related to inflammation and oxidative stress.

Alzheimer's disease affects 5-6 percent of the population above 60 years of age worldwide[215] and 10 percent of the American population over 65 years. The number in America is expected to quadruple by the year 2050. Because of its known anti-inflammatory and antioxidant effects, animal studies have been conducted on Alzheimer's disease and curcumin. In mice models, there was a 40-percent reduction in plaque in those mice treated with curcumin, which is an unbelievable reduction.[216] Notably, small doses over a long period of time were more effective than large doses in a short period of time, suggesting the benefit is long-term and the spice needs to be eaten over the long-term as well. Consider, then, the impact of eating turmeric over a lifetime.

Curcumin is also an important antiviral and antiseptic. For centuries, people have applied turmeric paste to cuts to prevent bacterial infections. It delivers important cardiovascular benefits as well: in studies on mice, fewer fatty deposits were found in those eating turmeric. Researchers also found notably less LDL and overall inflammation. [217] Similarly, a recent article compared rabbits which ate a high-cholesterol meal and turmeric with those who ate a high-cholesterol meal without the spice, and the rabbits which ate the added turmeric had less atherosclerotic plaque than their counterparts. The authors concluded that the effects of turmeric were multifaceted and included lowering both cholesterol and inflammatory markers.[218]

ROSEMARY: THE CANCER FIGHTER

HERBS, TOO, CAN BE IMPORTANT HEALTH-BOOSTERS, and one we love is rosemary. Rosemary has three essential components: rosemarinic acid, carnosic acid and carnosol. These elements are potent antioxidants. When we cook food on a grill at high temperatures and the food burns, it releases toxic chemicals called heterocyclic amines (HCAs). Traces of HCAs are found in breast, prostate and colon cancers. When we place rosemary on the grill with our food, studies show that the HCAs decrease. In a recent study, when rosemary extract was added to beef, HCA production was inhibited by 85-91 percent![219] Similarly, mice injected with carcinogens (cancer causing chemicals) who also received carnasol (component of rosemary) developed 61 percent fewer tumors. *(Consider 2)*

√ **CONSIDER 2**

Bring sprigs of rosemary to your next BBQ. Throw them onto the grill. They add great taste and help decrease cancer risk.

Rosemary has been around for centuries. There are references to it in the Bible. Early Greeks and Romans used it as a funeral decoration. Simply smelling rosemary has even been found to decrease cortisol (stress hormone). Rosemary is an important herb for its anti-cancer benefits, and it's one we try to use regularly in our diets.

CINNAMON: THE SWEETEST NON-SUGAR THAT HELPS LOWER SUGAR IN YOUR BLOOD

AS WE HAVE DISCUSSED, many chronic illnesses have become epidemic in modern society with less emphasis on exercise, sleep and good diet. Diabetes and cardiovascular disease are rampant.

Cinnamon is an important spice in treating diabetes; it's a good antioxidant and important in enhancing insulin sensitivity. Recall that in diabetes, the body does not respond to the insulin that is present, so sugar is not converted to fat—which is the main purpose of insulin. Sugar then circulates in the blood and becomes a risk for forming plaque in the heart. We have studies that show the benefits of adding cinnamon to foods to decrease blood sugars. When diabetic patients were given 1g, 3g or 6g of cinnamon, all groups showed improvement in blood sugar, triglycerides, LDL and total cholesterol compared to the control group. Interestingly, there was no dose-dependent relationship; meaning, it didn't matter whether people took 1g, 3g or 6g because they all experienced a significant, similar drop in sugar and cholesterol levels within about 40 days.[220]

People with diabetes, however, aren't the only ones who are rewarded for eating cinnamon. In one study, animals given high-fat/high-sugar diets and cinnamon were less likely to develop insulin resistance (i.e. pre-diabetes) than those not given the cinnamon.[221] This suggests that the benefits of cinnamon extend beyond treating diabetes, and can be useful in decreasing one's risk of *developing* diabetes as well.

Cinnamon is also a powerful antifungal agent.[222] It has antibacterial properties as well, with studies showing it's effective in combating molds, stomach bugs and common pneumonias.[223] Cinnamon is effective in killing oral bacteria—which is why we see cinnamon in chewing gum[224]—and it improves circulation and is a key ingredient in tiger balm, an herbal cream to ease sore joints. Another important benefit is its effect as an antioxidant. Small studies suggest that cinnamon oils can help remove free radicals, which are responsible for attacking our cells and creating cancers.[225] We also have data on cinnamon's ability to inhibit plaque formation in Alzheimer's disease. *(Consider 3)*

> √ **CONSIDER 3**
>
> Add cinnamon to your baked foods instead of sugar to sweeten. It actually lowers your sugar.

GARLIC: THE STINKING ROSE

GARLIC, THE "STINKING ROSE," is actually a vegetable but people often think of it as an herb. Historically, documents have been retrieved from 3500 years ago that claim garlic can be effective in treating heart disease.[226] Why is garlic so great? It's nutrient-rich: 65 percent water and the remainder is carbohydrates, protein, fiber and free amino acids. Garlic is loaded with potassium, phosphorus, zinc and selenium. It's known for its abundance of saponins, which are responsible for fighting against bacteria that might attack the plant. Like plants, which use saponins to fight off bacteria, we believe humans can harness the saponins and benefit from their antibacterial effects. Saponins are also believed to be effective anticancer treatments. *(Consider 4)*

> √ **CONSIDER 4**
>
> Add garlic to all your foods to help with heart disease. If you are coming down with a stomach bug think about adding garlic.

Phenols are antioxidants found in fruits, vegetables and spices. Garlic is rich in phenols so it is a potent antioxidant. Many studies have been done on garlic's lipid-lowering abilities. About half of the studies were negative but in the half that showed a benefit, the payoff was seen in people with the higher cholesterol levels. In those cases,

LDL cholesterol and triglycerides dropped by about 10 percent when they ate garlic.[227] Other studies show that in both normal subjects and those with high cholesterol, garlic works to block platelet aggregation. Recall, platelet aggregation can create plaque formation. Then garlic's healing qualities are similar to those of aspirin. [228] Further studies show that garlic also improves the elasticity of our blood vessels. Elasticity is a good thing because it allows blood vessels to change based on blood flow requirements.[229]

What kind of garlic is best? The answer is unclear. In the trials, many formulations were used. Some trials showed that aged garlic was superior but that isn't conclusive. Our bottom line is: eat garlic frequently because its benefits are short-acting. Don't worry so much about which garlic is better, just eat it. Fresh is always best.

OUR SPICE CABINET

DO WE KNOW OF MORE SPICES TO TALK ABOUT? Absolutely, but that will have to be a topic for another book! We just wanted to highlight some of the ones we really love, but on a daily basis, we try to get an abundance of spices into our diets. We regularly use cumin, coriander powder, pomegranate powder, ajowan (popular in Indian dishes), mango powder and black pepper. As you start your meal preparations, open your spice cupboard and consider which spices you could add to the recipe. ▪

YOUR PRESCRIPTION:
Finding the Spice of Your Life

❶ **Try to be creative by adding a little spice into all of your meals.** Try different combinations and experience the flavors.

❷ **Eat turmeric at least a few times each week. Add black pepper to help its absorption. Turmeric is super-important and should be used regularly.** It is bitter. Start by adding it to stews, beans, soups and then you will gradually become more comfortable with it. Now, we add it to our water. Flavor your water with it—add ½ tsp turmeric and 1/8 tsp ground black pepper to 20 ounces of water. Add a little lemon splash.

CHAPTER 11:

Water, The Essence of Life

Water is an integral part of our existence.

OUR BODIES ARE 60 PERCENT WATER. It is an essential component of the body's fluids, including blood, synovial fluid (fluid around the joints), saliva, digestive juices, lymph fluids, urine, sweat and tears. Water is also a part of every internal organ and system in the body. Those organs and systems need adequate water to operate effectively. The nervous system relies on fluids for communication. Our digestive system, lymph system and reproductive systems all rely on water for proper functioning. Every cell in our bodies needs water because water is the vehicle that distributes the electrolytes necessary for creating energy, transfers nutrients into cells and removes debris from the cells. Every bodily function requires water at some level.

Water is also critical for maintaining proper body temperature. When we feel hot, we sweat out water through our skin, and when it evaporates the body is able to cool itself. Sweating also is a form of detoxification. Water helps the stomach, eyes, mouth and throat stay moist by keeping the mucosal lining hydrated.

Every day, our bodies lose water through respiration (your foggy breath on a cold winter day), urination, sweating and fecal material, resulting in approximately 2.4 liters (just over 80 ounces) of water lost each and every day. Losses are then balanced by what we take in. We obtain our fluids from what we drink and the waters in our food. Water is the easiest way to hydrate our bodies. Water-rich fruits and vegetables are also great ways to keep hydrated.

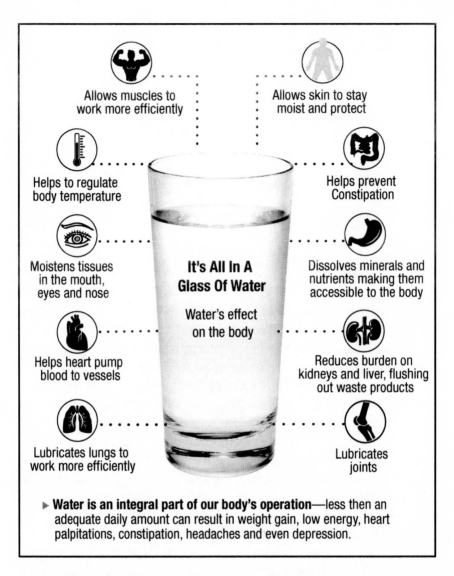

Allows muscles to work more efficiently

Allows skin to stay moist and protect

Helps to regulate body temperature

Helps prevent Constipation

Moistens tissues in the mouth, eyes and nose

It's All In A Glass Of Water

Water's effect on the body

Dissolves minerals and nutrients making them accessible to the body

Helps heart pump blood to vessels

Reduces burden on kidneys and liver, flushing out waste products

Lubricates lungs to work more efficiently

Lubricates joints

▶ **Water is an integral part of our body's operation**—less then an adequate daily amount can result in weight gain, low energy, heart palpitations, constipation, headaches and even depression.

When the brain detects that we lack water, it activates our thirst mechanism. If we don't quench our thirst, our urine becomes dark in color and our stool becomes hard and we become constipated. Without fluids, some people feel faint and lightheaded. Others get headaches. With longstanding dehydration, the kidneys start failing. People can develop palpitations (heart flutters), which resolve with fluid. We use hydration to maintain blood pressure.

A dehydrated body is a stressed body, and stress is a major source of disease. A healthy body can live for several weeks without food, but it cannot survive more than several days without some water. Severe dehydration for an extended time can kill you. Many people do not understand that coffee, sodas, juices and many energy drinks have a dehydrating effect on the body and do not replenish our bodies. Sodas, tea, coffee and juices are not good options for hydration because they have so many other ingredients. The sugars in juice and caffeine in tea cause us to urinate without actually hydrating us. Most people simply do not consume enough water and high-water-content foods.

> √ **CONSIDER 1**
>
> ▪ When you're hungry try drinking a glass of water before you start eating something.
>
> ▪ People can confuse dehydration with hunger—drinking a glass of water can dissipate our desire to eat.

Dehydration also can contribute to weight gain and obesity. People often confuse dehydration with hunger. Often, when we feel our stomachs grumbling, we reach for food when in fact, we are simply thirsty and need to drink some water. People also choose to consume high-caloric drinks such as sodas, fruit juices and energy drinks instead of water, adding to weight gain. Our metabolisms will actually slow down when we are dehydrated, thus burning fewer calories, again raising the potential for weight gain.[230] (*Consider 1*)

Many of our clients are successful in changing their food choices and they start losing unwanted weight. Then, suddenly they become frustrated because they're eating nutritious whole foods and exercising, but their weight loss has stopped before they've reached their goals.

Why does this happen? Often, people's diet diaries reveal that they aren't drinking enough water. Amazingly enough, simply drinking enough water gets them back on track for their weight loss goals. (*Consider 2*)

People often ask about the optimal amount to drink, but no one

> √ **CONSIDER 2**
>
> Coffee, sodas, juices and energy drinks have a dehydrating effect on the body
>
> ❶ What percent of your daily liquid intake is actually water versus other beverages?
>
> ❷ Try tracking the number of glasses of water you drink in one day. Note: a glass holds almost 2 cups of water—*Some experts believe you should drink 8 cups (64 ounces) of water per day.*

really knows the answer. Some experts say we should drink eight cups of water per day. We don't really know if that is the best quantity, and many believe that even more would be beneficial. People complain, though, that they have to go to the bathroom too often when they drink enough water—but urinating frequently is a good thing. Remember, your kidneys are excreting toxins in your urine, so it is good to go to the bathroom more often; just keep an eye on the color of the urine and gauge if you are drinking enough.

So our recommendations is to drink water often and in larger quantities. Avoid sodas and juices, which are empty calories and don't hydrate you. If you enjoy tea and coffee, understand that you're not hydrating and drink water along with your caffeinated drinks. Your goal should be to urinate every two hours. There is no recommended amount of water to drink. Listen to your body. Listen to your thirst. Get yourself a 20-ounce bottle, fill it full of water and drink the entire bottle, three to four times a day. You will be refreshed. ▪

YOUR PRESCRIPTION:

❶ **Drink water often** and in fairly large amounts each day.

❷ **There is no substitute** for water.

❸ **Think about when you urinated last.** Has it been a while? You should try to urinate once every couple of hours. Look at your urine. If it is dark, you need to go back and drink more water.

CHAPTER 12:

Sleep On It

Rejuvenate and detoxify by

catching some ZZZZs

D R. RAO: *When my third child was just five weeks old, I received a frantic phone call from my older son's second-grade teacher. The teacher had noticed an issue with my son over the past three weeks and she was concerned. He had become easily distracted, was not following directions and not completing classwork assignments, which was a big departure from the past. She felt he was showing signs of ADHD and recommended that I seek medical attention for him.*

The following week, my son picked up a soccer ball in the middle of a game when he was not playing the goalie position. This concerned his coach, who had worked with him for three years. My husband and I were starting to worry about these new distractible symptoms and, feeling very frustrated, my husband asked, "What is wrong with you?" Our son replied with equal frustration in his voice, "It's not like I have slept since the baby was born!" It was then I realized my son was suffering from poor sleep because of the daily disruptions from the baby. He hadn't had a good night's sleep in weeks. We moved my son to another bedroom so he couldn't hear the baby crying at night and the very next day, he woke up refreshed and feeling like himself again. Within days, his concentration and strange behavior had resolved.

SLEEP: IT'S NOT JUST ABOUT BEING TIRED

S IEEP DISORDERS AFFECT 50 to 70 million Americans. Unfortunately, inadequate sleep is common in our society. The most obvious symptom is daytime fatigue; over time it can cause a depressed mood, irritability and poor concentration. Lack of sleep can also lead to difficulty with weight loss and metabolic issues such as diabetes and hypertension. In addition, it also has a significant impact on the person's safety. Those who sleep less than eight hours are two to four times as likely to be involved in a car crash.[231] The National Sleep Foundation recommends that adults aged 18 to 64 get between seven and nine hours of restorative sleep in order to maintain health.[232]

As early as the 18th century, it was understood that there was a cyclical nature to a day that was 24 hours long and corresponds to the Earth's rotation. This rotation also connects to the biological clock in our cells, leading to a circadian rhythm. Circadian rhythms are the biological, physical and behavioral changes that occur with a 24-hour sleep/wake cycle. The circadian rhythm is set to environmental cues such as the rising and setting of the sun. Researchers have more recently discovered that hormones such as cortisol (that stress hormone again) also are affected by that same cycle. Recall, cortisol is our "wake up" hormone; it takes cues from external sources such as sunlight and is at its peak in the early morning.

During daylight hours, we have higher levels of cortisol. These levels subside as the day progresses, and as cortisol wanes, levels of adenosine and melatonin increase. Adenosine is a chemical that increases during the day and promotes sleepiness as the day goes on. As evening approaches and the light disappears, melatonin also increases and prepares our body for sleep. Melatonin is often considered our "sleep hormone" because it works to synchronize our biological clocks. Melatonin is released when it gets dark, and the amount in our system peaks at around 2-4 a.m. On the other hand, when we are asleep, our bodies break down adenosine and it drops to a low level in the morning. Low levels of adenosine promote wakefulness. Since we know that melatonin promotes sleeping, it makes sense that people take melatonin supplements to regulate their sleep.

With sleep debt, cortisol breaks down more slowly. Therefore, when we don't sleep, these stress hormones remain at a higher level. Recall that higher levels of stress hormones (chronic distress) over time can lead to inflammation. More on this later.

HOW MUCH SLEEP DO WE NEED?

SLEEP REQUIREMENTS CHANGE AS WE AGE. Newborns sleep most of the time—16-18 hours per day. As they reach the toddler stage, children sleep 11-13 hours and need frequent naps. According to the National Sleep Foundation, children require from 10-13 hours in their younger years (ages 3-5) and by the time they become pre-teens they need 9-11 hours of sleep.

When children become teenagers, they still require 8-10 hours of sleep per night. How many of our high school students actually sleep that much, given their late nights and early wake-up alarms? Adults and seniors require 7-9 hours of sleep per day. Do you get enough sleep? Does is matter if you don't? [234] *(Figure 1) (Consider 1)*

> ## CONSIDER ❶
>
> √ **Do you get enough sleep?**
>
> √ **How many hours would you sleep if the alarm did not wake you up?**
>
> √ **Do you feel rested when you wake up?**

STAGES OF SLEEP

IN A NORMAL CYCLE, we go through several stages of sleep—one stage of REM (rapid eye movement) and four stages of Non-REM sleep. REM sleep is a time of low muscle tone and rapid eye move-

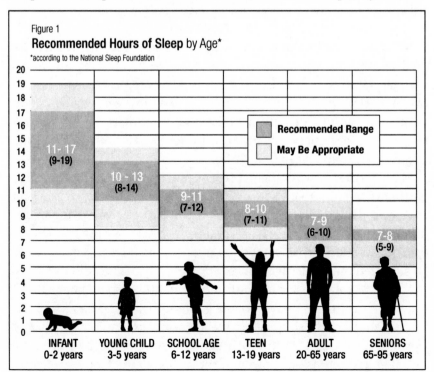

Figure 1
Recommended Hours of Sleep by Age*
*according to the National Sleep Foundation

INFANT 0-2 years	YOUNG CHILD 3-5 years	SCHOOL AGE 6-12 years	TEEN 13-19 years	ADULT 20-65 years	SENIORS 65-95 years
11-17 (9-19)	10-13 (8-14)	9-11 (7-12)	8-10 (7-11)	7-9 (6-10)	7-8 (5-9)

Recommended Range
May Be Appropriate

ments. This cycle lasts about 90 minutes and recurs frequently through the night. The REM sleep cycle increases in length as sleep continues through the night. REM sleep is the time when people dream the most vividly. About 50 percent of a baby's sleeping hours are REM, but for adults REM time shrinks to about 20 percent. The full benefit of these individual stages is not entirely clear but we do know that all stages are necessary. Restorative sleep requires four to five cycles of all stages of Non-REM and REM sleep. If we don't get that sleep, we call that sleep debt, which can be associated with multiple health issues which will be discussed.

Seniors in general struggle with sleep and often suffer from sleep debt. Along with the physical changes that occur as we get older, changes to our sleep patterns are a part of the normal aging process. As people age, they tend to have a harder time falling asleep and more trouble staying asleep than when they were younger. However, it is a common misconception that as we age, we need less sleep. In fact, research demonstrates that our sleep needs remain constant throughout adulthood. So, what's keeping seniors awake? Often, it is a mechanical problem such as need to urinate, medication side effect or a complication of a physical/psychiatric illness. Interestingly, though, older people spend more time in the lighter stages of sleep than in deep sleep.

Many older adults also report being less satisfied with sleep and more tired during the day. Studies on the sleep habits of older Americans show an increase in the time it takes to fall asleep (sleep latency), an overall decline in REM sleep, and an increase in sleep fragmentation (waking up during the night) with age. Naps during the day may work to eliminate sleepiness, but they cannot reverse all of the detrimental effects of disruptive sleep.

Many modern environmental factors provoke sleep debt. First, some of us have to work night shifts several times a week. Shift work or any other forced change in our clocks, such as being caregivers at night, can disrupt our circadian rhythms. We also travel, often for work, at all hours of the day to places in different time zones. We are then forced to operate on a different time clock without any opportunity to restore our systems.

Many of us stay up late to finish chores or just get some "alone time" before we turn in. We have trouble going to bed at 10 p.m., in order to get eight hours of sleep before the alarm wakes us at 6 a.m. Most of us check emails and social media late into the night. Then there are the late-night television shows and shows previously taped. Even after we're asleep, our tables and phones buzz all night and interrupt our rest. Does this sound familiar? To most of us, it does. All of these activities impact our natural circadian rhythm. The unnatural light lowers our melatonin levels. *(Consider 2)*

Medical illnesses can also create sleep debt. Neurodegenerative conditions such as dementia, Parkinson's disease, pain, anxiety and depression can cause sleep interruption. Benign prostate hypertrophy (BPH), a benign condition which causes the prostate gland to enlarge in men and as a result causes frequent urination, or pelvic floor weakening in women (after multiple children) also deprive us of sleep. Menopause, too, is often associated with sleep disruption. Sleep apnea, which causes a person to stop breathing at night for short periods, causes disrupted sleep as the body wakes up to breathe. Certain medications such as antidepressants also can act like stimulants, which increase nighttime arousal. Stimulants such as caffeine, tea, chocolate and sodas can keep our systems activated for up to eight hours and thus, prevent us from calming down enough to sleep. Nicotine from cigarettes also can keep us activated late into the night. *(Consider 3)*

> ## CONSIDER
>
> √ **How late do you check your email?**
>
> √ **What is the last thing you do before you sleep?**
>
> √ **Is your mind racing because you just watched the news or due to an email that you just read?**

SLEEP AND OUR STRESS HORMONES: THE LINK BETWEEN STRESS AND CORTISOL

EARLIER WE MENTIONED that cortisol levels should be highest in the morning and decrease throughout the day. During the evening, we have higher levels of adenosine and melatonin which help us sleep. Sleep deprivation has a major impact on stress hormone regulation through two pathways: activity at the brain level and through the autonomic nervous system—the nervous system in charge of our stress response.

The pituitary gland is considered the master endocrine gland and con-

> ## CONSIDER
>
> √ **Do you have trouble sleeping at night?**
>
> √ **Do you take in any stimulants like tea, coffee, or chocolate in the afternoon?**

Figure 2:

THE STRESS OF NOT SLEEPING

Cortisol and Sleep Debt

SLEEP DEBT:

❶ **Activates Sympathetic Nervous System** ▷ Increase adrenaline ▷ Makes us feel wired

❷ **Inhibits Parasympathetic Nervous System** ▷ Decrease ability to rest and digest

❸ **Activates prolonged elevated levels of Cortisol** ▷ Increases inflammatory markers

---

trols secretion of several hormones. During normal sleep patterns, our growth hormone is released, emphasizing the need for better sleep in order to grow. Normally, while we sleep, cortisol production is decreased. When sleep deprivation occurs, however, it causes a stress response and the sympathetic nervous system (fight-or-flight) is activated.[235] Our adrenaline increases and we are ready to get moving. With chronic sleep deprivation, our hormone balance is disrupted. One study illustrates this concept. It looked at eleven men who slept 4-6 hours per night and noted that those with this sleep debt had higher evening cortisol levels and higher activation of the sympathetic nervous system than their counterparts who slept more.[236]

Sleep debt, then, is a distress to our bodies (see chapter 4), similar to chronic stress. We see increases in our inflammatory markers with sleep debt as well (tumor necrosis factor and Interleukin 6).[237] These markers are part of our immune system defense and respond to enemies such as viral infections and tumors. They

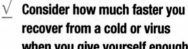

CONSIDER ❹

√ **Consider how much faster you recover from a cold or virus when you give yourself enough time to sleep**

help the body fight foreign cells by creating symptoms such as a fever and recruiting other fighter cells into the areas where there is inflammation—A GOOD THING. However, in the presence of chronic inflammation from persistent sleep loss, these markers can be persistently elevated and cause symptoms of fatigue and sluggishness—A BAD THING. *(Figure 2), (Consider 4)*

SLEEP AS AN ANTIOXIDANT

ANOTHER VERY IMPORTANT ASPECT OF SLEEP is its antioxidant potential. In order for the body to work, it needs oxygen. However, the use of oxygen in cellular reactions can generate free radicals which make our cells unstable and cause damage to our DNA. Consequently, this can lead to chronic illness including a nidus for cancer-causing cells. Multiple triggers for this free radical formation have been discussed in previous chapters. Antioxidants are needed to protect our cells against damage from this oxidative stress. Sleep deprivation adversely affects the immune system and creates even higher oxidative stress and in turn contributes to even more metabolic imbalances. [238, 239] In contrast, sleep is restorative and serves as an antioxidant.

Glutathione, produced by the liver, is one of the strongest antioxidants in our bodies. We've learned that as little as five days of sleep deprivation can impair the production of glutathione by 30 percent,[240] and studies show that a glutathione depletion of 20-30 percent can impair cellular defense systems and lead to abnormal cell-to-cell communication, cause adverse effects to protein breakdown and cell injury.[241] In an animal study, sleep deprivation accelerated glutathione depletion which showed an increase in cell damage in heart tissue. However, sleep recovery showed the restoration and antioxidant activity in both liver and heart. [242]

It has been shown that the immune system works best if there are balanced levels of glutathione. This has been studied most extensively in patients with HIV (human immunodeficiency virus) infection where there is a severe immune system dysfunction due to the virus attacking the immune T lymphocyte cells. In the studies, those patients taking glutathione like compounds had significant increases in their immunological functions.[243] More research is needed but this maybe another reason we see immune dysfunction (increase colds) with sleep deprivation. *(Consider 5)*

> ## CONSIDER
>
> √ Glutathione has a sulfur group on it which makes it a very effective antioxidant.
>
> √ Consider that getting restful sleep may help keep your glutathione levels up.
>
> √ Foods high in sulfur group are garlic, onions, cruciferous vegetables such as broccoli, kale, collards, cabbage, cauliflower.

SLEEP DEBT AND PERFORMANCE

IMPAIRED PERFORMANCE CAN AFFECT your personal safety, as well as efficiency at work or play. As we sleep less and become more sleep deprived, our diminished alertness translates into more workplace errors and higher numbers of auto accidents with drivers falling asleep at the wheel.[244]

Studies have looked at daytime alertness in the workplace as well. Dr. David Dinges, head of the Sleep and Chronology Laboratory at the University of Pennsylvania, divided dozens of people into three groups: those who slept for four hours, six hours and eight hours for a two-week period. He did psychomotor testing, which involved subjects' performing simple tasks such as pressing a space bar of a computer when they noted a certain symbol on the computer. He found that those people who slept eight hours had no difficulty with their psychomotor testing, whereas both the four-hour and six-hour sleep groups showed significant declines in their psychomotor performance over the two-week period.[245]

At the halfway point of the study, 25 percent of the six-hour group was falling asleep at the computer. They had trouble with basic math questions and cognitive skills. By the end of the study, performance reduced significantly. The New York Times article about the study read, "Six-hour sleepers were as impaired as those who, in another Dinges study, had been sleep–deprived for 24 hours straight—the cognitive equivalent of being legally drunk."[246, 247] It was noted that seven hours was not enough sleep and cognitive testing was impaired even at that level of sleep. This sleep deprivation is what Dr. Rao believed affected her son's behavior. In fact, older studies show that if we reduce our sleep for even one night by 1.3 to 1.5 hours, our daytime alertness is decreased by 32 percent.[248] *(Consider 6)*

> ## CONSIDER ⑥
>
> 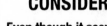 **Even though it seems we can get more done by staying awake longer** and taking that time out of our sleep, our efficiency the next day can be reduced by 32 percent. You will be better off to save the work to tomorrow and get a good night sleep

SLEEP DEBT AND DISEASE

STUDIES ARE MOUNTING SHOWING that short sleep periods, poor sleep quality and sleep deprivation are associated with diabetes, metabolic syndrome and obesity.[249, 250, 251] This can be attributed to several issues, including hormones affected by poor sleep. Insulin is one hormone that regulates glucose metabolism, or the process of using sugar for energy. Sleep deprivation for as little as a week has been shown to cause changes in the body which can mimic the insulin resistance seen in Type 2 diabetes.[252, 253]

In one study, fasting morning glucose in those experiencing sleep debt (4h) was 15 points higher than those who had slept normally.[254] In other words, if you had slept for only four hours, your fasting sugar in the morning was 15 points higher than those who had slept for eight hours. Remember, fasting blood sugar is used to diagnose diabetes. Fifteen points can absolutely make a difference in whether you have the disease or you don't. As discussed in Chapter 5, high blood sugar levels eventually lead to insulin resistance, which then can cause diabetes.

When we sleep less, it may actually shorten our lifespan! *(Consider 7)* In an observational study, men who slept for fewer than six hours lived a shorten lifespan than those who slept more. (This was adjusted for hypertension and diabetes.)[255] There also appears to be a higher incidence of other cardiovascular risk factors in sleep-deprived people such as hypertension, obesity, diabetes, heart disease and stroke.[256] These illnesses are likely triggered by the inflammation caused by sleep debt.

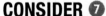

CONSIDER ❼

√ When you sleep less, you can potentially shorten your lifespan.

APPETITE AND SLEEP

OUR APPETITE FOR HIGH-CALORIE FOODS also increases with sleep deprivation. That trend is partly due to your body's extra demands for calories and energy, simply because you are awake longer. Several hormones associated with weight management also get affected. Ghrelin is a hormone, secreted by the stomach, which stimulates appetite and has been shown to increase with sleep loss. Therefore, you are more hungry when you sleep less. Leptin is the hormone that tells your body that it is full and your appetite decreases. After only two nights of sleep deprivation (4 h), ghrelin production increased by 28 percent and leptin production decreased by 18 percent.[257] In other words, two days of sleeping four hours makes you hungrier and reduces your body's ability to know you are full.

Sleep loss also changes how we utilize energy. One study showed that sleep deprivation slowed down fat loss by 55 percent compared to a control group with similar caloric intake.[258] This may be one reason why so many sleep-deprived people are unable to lose weight in spite of restricting their calories. *(Figure 3)*

SLEEP DEBT AND MEMORY

THE ACT OF LEARNING NEW INFORMATION requires several pathways within the hippocampus, a part of our brain critical for memory. When we make memories, we perceive smell, taste and feelings, and these sensations are transmitted to the hippocampus and integrated. It's believed that in the hippocampus, it is decided if something perceived is worth remembering. With sleep debt, disruptions to the pathways to the hippocampus have been noted, so our memories aren't as sharp.[259]

As early as 1924, studies were done showing that retention of nonsense syllables and short stories was better with sleep than without. Many studies since have shown that sleep debt causes difficulty in memory recall. How much sleep and what stages of sleep are required for memory are unclear. Some more recent studies have shown that we need more non-REM sleep for memories of stories, words and random information. You'll remember that non-REM sleep is sleep that usually occurs at the beginning of the night. Storing of emotional memories, however, appears to require more REM sleep, which occurs later in the evening.[260]

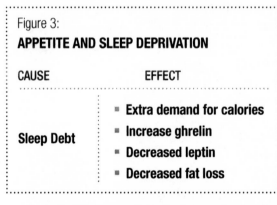

Figure 3:
APPETITE AND SLEEP DEPRIVATION

CAUSE	EFFECT
Sleep Debt	▪ Extra demand for calories ▪ Increase ghrelin ▪ Decreased leptin ▪ Decreased fat loss

Cortisol plays a role in making memories as well. We know that during early parts of sleep, cortisol levels are at their lowest. It appears that low levels of cortisol are needed for storing memories. In studies where patients were either given hydrocortisone (a cortisol like compound) or had high levels of cortisol due to a medical illness, notable impairments in word recall and memory related were noted. [261] We also know that with sleep debt, cortisol does not break down well. Consider this cycle then: when we are stressed, we have higher cortisol levels. With higher cortisol, we have more trouble sleeping. With higher cortisol, we have less ability to retain memories.

SLEEP APNEA

SLEEP APNEA ALSO TRIGGERS MEMORY LOSS.[262] Sleep apnea is characterized by heavy snoring and intermittent episodes of apnea, or absence of breathing. During those times of not breathing, less oxygen gets to the brain and organs. The body realizes the problem and causes the person to wake up, leading to significant sleep disruption. However, the person then falls back to sleep and has more episodes of apnea. The cycle repeats itself, over and over during the night.

Apnea is associated with hypertension and headaches, and higher rates of stroke, heart disease, abnormal heart rhythms and heart failure. Sleep apnea directly impacts and alters endothelial function as well.[263] Recall that the endothelial cells are the cells that line our blood vessels; damage to these cells results in the cascade of inflammation and oxidative stress. The blood vessel also becomes impaired and can't open as well in response to more demand for blood.

CASE 1: 50 year old male *who was noted to have daytime fatigue and high CRP (marker of inflammation) elevated to 43 (normal is up to 3). He had known sleep apnea but was having trouble wearing his mask. He also had been working the night shift for the past 5 years. He shifted his night shift to day shift and started wearing his CPAP for his sleep apnea regularly. In 6 weeks, his CRP returned to normal range.*

Drops in oxygen levels with sleep apnea can lead to shrinking of cells in our brains (mammillary bodies), which are involved with our memory and thinking. Diminished mammillary body volume in OSA patients may be associated with memory and spatial orientation deficits found in the syndrome. The mechanisms contributing to the volume loss are unclear, but may relate to hypoxic/ischemic processes (low oxygen states), possibly assisted by nutritional deficiencies in the syndrome.[264]

Sleep apnea most commonly occurs in people who are overweight. It

---

CONSIDER

√ **Talk to your provider about getting a sleep study if you answer yes to some or all of these questions:**

1. Have you been noted to have daytime sleepiness?

2. Do you snore?

3. Do you have uncontrolled blood pressure or a BMI of greater than 35?

can continue to make attempted weight loss more difficult. Why? Sleep apnea can lower the metabolism, which makes weight loss challenging. Reversing sleep apnea not only improves daytime fatigue but it also can rev up your metabolism, making it easier to lose weight. It also can reverse many of the cardiovascular risk factors and risks for other chronic inflammatory diseases. *(Consider 8)*

WHAT ABOUT SLEEP DEBT AND CANCER?

SLEEP DEPRIVATION HAS BEEN ASSOCIATED with increased risk for cancers. Studies show a relationship of sleep to the hormone melatonin. Melatonin, along with promoting sleep, has been shown to inhibit cancer development and growth, and improve immune our function. It also has an antioxidant effect.[265]

Some believe that sleep disturbance leads to immune suppression, which results in cancer-promoting cytokines. These cytokines are molecules which help with cell to cell communication in immune responses and help mobilize cells to move to sites where there is inflammation. One study in Denmark showed a 1.5-fold increase in risk for primary breast cancer among women who worked mostly at night for at least six months. They also produced more cytokines, presumably because they didn't experience enough darkness. Without the darkness, they didn't produce enough melatonin to power their immune systems properly and cytokines developed.[266, 267] It is hypothesized that melatonin is regulated by the retina in the back of the eyes which recognizes light and darkness. Women who are blind and cannot detect light—and as a result their melatonin levels are not inhibited—have a 50-percent lower relative risk of breast cancer than women who can "see" light.[268]

Even weak light during nighttime decreases our melatonin production. Changing working hours isn't always something we can control, but working on reducing ambient light by turning off email, reading print books rather than reading on a tablet or other electronic device and not watching TV at night, can not only improve our sleep but may lower our risk of certain cancers as well.

BLUE LIGHT

STUDIES HAVE LOOKED AT THE ROLE of electronics and brain wave chemistry at bedtime and its effect on melatonin. A 2014 study published in The Proceedings of the National Academy of Sciences showed that reading from an electronic book instead of a traditional book increased the time needed to fall asleep because of reduced drowsiness. Further, melatonin levels of those in the study were lower in the blood at night, and people were less alert in the morning than those who read a paper book.[269]

In pre-industrial times, our cues for circadian rhythm were based on sunlight. The pineal gland in our brains releases melatonin rhythmically, with levels peaking during the "dark period" at night.[270] However, our use of alternative light sources sends signals to our retina, stimulating our photosensitive retinal ganglion cells, also called ipRGCs, which can detect ambient light information and signal our brains to cut back on our melatonin production.[271] These cells have a crude ability to pick up light, so a night light or a light placed far from us, usually will not impact these changes. It is the bigger items—our electronics, lights on in rooms—that affect our melatonin levels. Also, it turns out that these cells are most sensitive to blue light, which is what most tablets use.[272]

> ## CONSIDER ⑨
>
> √ You can decrease the alertness caused by your devices by using a filter with your device, dimming the light and holding your device farther away from your eyes

Mariana Figueiro of the Rensselaer Polytechnic Institute has done extensive research on these changes.[273] She also found out that blue light leads to a faster heart rate and causes EEG changes (brain wave changes), which show increased beta waves and correspond to increased alertness. You can avoid this by using a filter with your device, dimming the light or holding your device farther away from your eyes. (Consider 9)

> ## CONSIDER ⑩
>
> √ Challenge yourself to turn off your electronics 1 to 2 hours prior to bedtime? Too much? Ok, then start smaller and try increasing it in increments of 30 minutes .

CRAZY THOUGHT

WE BELIEVE THE ONE HOUR of "productive work" you get at the very end of the day is often negated by the sluggishness and decreased alertness you experience in the morning. We think we all should learn to shut down our electronics at least two hours before bedtime. We realize that in our global economy, there is always daylight in some part of the world and some professions expect a 24/7 approach. However, if you look at it from a productivity perspective, the science shows, restful sleep leads to better performance and longevity. *(Consider 10)*

TEENS

ONE OF OUR BIGGEST CONCERNS is the lack of sleep among teens. The circadian rhythm in teens is different from that of adults: they tend to be night owls and their rhythms shift towards a melatonin surge later in the evening. They also are more sensitive to blue light than adults which adds to the daytime drowsiness brought on by their early school schedules. The American Pediatric Association recommends 8.5 to 10 hours for sleep for teenagers, but fewer than 50 percent of American teens get that sleep. A University of Minnesota Study showed that those high schools that moved their start times to 8:30 a.m. have noticed improved grades in school and achievement tests, better attendance rates and reduced car accident rates. Other studies show that better sleep translates into better behavior and mood in adolescents.[274] *(Consider 11)*

> ## CONSIDER ⑪
> √ If our children are allowed to sleep without interruption when would they naturally wake up?

LEARNING/DETOXIFICATION

HOW DOES SLEEP REFRESH US? Scientists have shown through animal trials that our brain cells can shrink during sleep, which allows for increase in interstitial space, or space between cells. They further observed that during this sleep time, the fluid between the cells and the cerebrospinal fluid, which bathes our nerve tissue, increases the rate of removal and clearance of proteins such as B amyloid and other neurotoxins (toxins for the brain). Their findings suggest that sleep, more than wakefulness, more effectively removes our waste products or detoxifies our brains after a day of activity.

Dr. Barbara Oakley, a professor of engineering at Oakland University, teaches courses on learning and feels that sleep is critical to learning new material. She states, "This nightly housecleaning is part of what keeps your brain healthy. When you get too little sleep, the buildup of these toxic products is believed to explain why you cannot think very clearly." She highlights the role of sleep in learning and creativity in her book, A Mind for Numbers, and in her free online course called "Learning How to Learn."[275] She reports that falling asleep while thinking about difficult concepts can help cement the learning processes for new ideas and concepts. Examples of famous intellectuals who used sleep to formulate new ideas were Thomas Edison and Salvador Dali; both got into mindsets that were very relaxed and eventually they drifted off to sleep. Some historians believe they discovered new ways to approach their tough problems using this technique, and were able to think of creative solutions when they awoke.

People often wear sleep deprivation as a badge of honor on their sleeves. Some correlate it with improved efficiency, and "excess" sleep has at times been equated with laziness as well. However, if you look at it with productivity in mind, the science shows, restful sleep leads to better performance and longevity. In addition, research has shown that sleep deprivation increases our sympathetic overdrive, decreases healing and reduces important hormones such as growth hormone. Further, sleep deprivation impairs our memory, leads to glucose imbalances, reduces our ability to detox and leads to weight gain. Along with decreased reaction time, higher risk for accidents, inhibiting creativity and worsening mood, sleep deprivation leaves you with much more than just being tired: sleep deprivation also increases your risk of chronic disease.

Not convinced? Why don't you sleep on it? (Figure 4) ▪

Figure 4:
SLEEP HYGIENE
adapted from the National Sleep Foundation:

Practices that can help you get a good night's sleep:

- Exercise can promote good sleep but some people can have a hard time falling asleep when they exercise at night because of the endorphin—adrenalin release. And so exercise, but exercise early

- Avoid food too close to bedtime, especially if you have issues with heartburn

- Keep room dark during the night

- Try to get natural light during the day

- Switch off your electronics 1-2 hours before bed

YOUR PRESCRIPTION:

1 **Try to work towards sleeping the goal allotment** for your age. Add 15 minutes of sleep each week and build up. Whatever it is can wait till morning

2 **Avoid looking at your electronics for 1-2 hours prior to bed.** Too hard? Start with 30 minutes

3 **When you lay down and your mind is racing, start taking deep breaths**. Focus on your breath. Take ten deep breaths. Exhale twice as long as you inhale. Bet you won't make to ten ;)

CHAPTER 13:

The Mind-Body Connection

Unleash the healing power of a calm mind

**CASE 1: A 50-YEAR-OLD MALE WHO WAS 100 POUNDS OVER-
WEIGHT**, *a photographer and videographer, came to our office. He had a
history of knee pain, diabetes and high cholesterol. Due to his knee pain and
fatigue, he led a mostly sedentary life. Two years ago, he started a weekly
Bikram yoga class in order to spend more time with his girlfriend. Bikram
yoga is a type of yoga where poses are done under high heat and humidity to
trigger a significant sweat response. He had difficulty staying in the class for
the first few sessions due to the excessive heat. But, each class he did a little
more. He stayed with the classes and noticed they gave him more energy and
cleared his mind. He realized that he wanted to make better food choices and,
as his muscle strength grew, he was able to increase activity outside the class.
He then added cycling to his regimen.*

*Over the next two years, he lost 100 pounds, came off most of his pain
medications, and his metabolic issues diminished. He continues to lead an
active lifestyle. At present, he continues his yoga, along with the other cardiovascular exercises. The yoga makes him feel peaceful, he says, and improves his creativity. His arthritis is gone. His diabetes and high cholesterol
have resolved.*

CASE 2: A 50-YEAR-OLD MALE EXECUTIVE *came in for a physical
exam. His travel and meeting schedule did not allow him to fast properly
for blood work or show up for his appointment. He had to reschedule his
visit three times in three months due to urgent conflicts. During the entire*

appointment, his phone vibrated with new texts and calls. It turned out his cardiovascular testing and fitness was normal but his stress parameters on a questionnaire and adaptability to stress were very abnormal.

Upon further questioning, he reported that he was feeling intense stress all of the time. His business was extremely successful and he had an active, supportive family; however, he constantly worried about the next steps for his business. His health was stable at the time of his visit, but we wondered how he would do after five to ten years of this constant stress? We wondered what tools we could provide him to calm himself.

Does this sound like you or someone else you know, who multitasks all day? How many of us have been in a situation where we have had to take on much more on our plate for several weeks or months? You look back and say to yourself, "How did I ever manage that?" Well, it was your acute stress response and adaptation. During such times, it's important to eat nutrient-rich foods with high levels of antioxidants, and rest well to be able to sustain yourself. After it is over, you need a period to recharge yourself (activation of the parasympathetic nervous system). After using all the gas, we have to go to the refilling station. If we don't refill, recharge, refresh, we break down, just like our cars. Our bodies break down, too.

But how do we reduce our stress? How do we learn to calm down? Sometimes, this is easier said than done. Sometimes it is hard to shut off the stimuli and slow down, no question. But what if you had a tool to improve your sense of peace, reduce the dread and anxiety of the stress, lower the inflammation and oxidative stress and improve restorative sleep before, during and after the stress was over?

MIND/BODY

WHEN WE WERE IN MEDICAL SCHOOL, we were told treatments for certain illnesses were "lifestyle changes." Those changes were usually summed up as eating a good diet, exercising and reducing stress. Ask most physicians and they can't explain what lifestyle changes truly means because the truth is, we aren't taught how to make those lifestyle changes in medical school. We know that sleep is important but weren't taught how to aid sleep. We know that exercise is important but weren't taught what exercises to give our patients. And we certainly were not taught techniques for reducing stress in medical school.

We learned these tools from personal experience and then we started going back to the data. We now teach our patients how to decrease stress. These tools are often called mind/body techniques and they encompass yoga, exercise postures, breathing techniques and meditation. Studies show how such techniques help suppress sympathetic overdrive and increase the rest and recovery function of the parasympathetic nervous system.[276] These techniques help us refill our tanks.

Let's start with yoga. Yoga, which literally means to add or connect, gives us a method for uniting the mind, body and spirit. It has been used to describe many things: breathing techniques (pranayama), postures (asana), and meditative practices, or a combination of these techniques. We will discuss each of these as different concepts so that we can understand the individual components *(Figure 1)*.

Yoga has been shown to lower inflammation and recharge our nervous system. It can be a unique practice tailored to each individual and can be done without leaving your home. It is a healing modality that does not need an appointment, and once the techniques are learned, it can be free of charge.

Often when we mention yoga to patients, they picture an image of a contortionist. However, the most beneficial parts of yoga can even be done sitting upright in a chair or lying down for a guided meditation. Yoga can be many things to many people. It is a discipline that allows for promotion of peace or calming of mind and strengthening of the body.

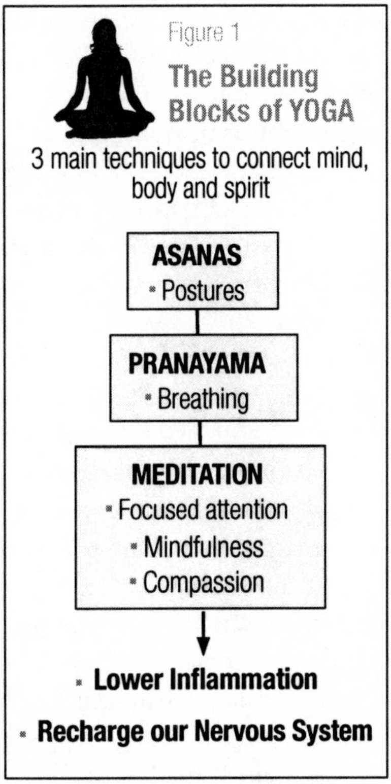

Figure 1

The Building Blocks of YOGA

3 main techniques to connect mind, body and spirit

ASANAS
* Postures

PRANAYAMA
* Breathing

MEDITATION
* Focused attention
* Mindfulness
* Compassion

* **Lower Inflammation**
* **Recharge our Nervous System**

HISTORY OF YOGA

YOGA ORIGINATED IN THE EAST. It is seen on artifacts dating back 5,000 years and is commented on in some of the earliest religious texts. In these references, yoga was seen as a tool to create harmony. Initially, it was meant for community wellness before it became an individual regimen. Highly spiritual leaders would guide people in ritual and ceremony to overcome the limitations of the mind. In these early texts, yogic practice was noted to also have meditation. People would focus on the lotus pose that the Buddha used in order to achieve enlightenment.

Over the centuries, yoga has transformed from ceremonies and meditation to more about fixed postures. In the 19th century, yoga was introduced in the West by Swami Vivekananda at the World Parliament of Religions in Chicago. His speech on eastern tradition and yoga was received with a standing ovation. At the time, the focus of yoga was on health and vegetarianism. After this, more and more Eastern influence made its way to America. In 1920, Paramahansa Yogananda, author of Autobiography of a Yogi (which is a classic in spiritual literature), spoke at a religious conference in Boston.[277] This event triggered a fascination with Eastern culture in using yogic postures as a health tool. By the 1960s, Maharishi Mahesh popularized Transcendental meditation.

WHAT IS YOGA TODAY?

THERE ARE NUMEROUS TYPES OF YOGA, which can make it confusing and overwhelming to begin a practice. As you will see, however, any yoga practices can offer incredible health benefits.

Yoga can be broken down into many different styles. One common style of yoga seen in the U.S. is Hatha yoga. Hatha yoga is an umbrella term for the practice which utilizes asanas or poses in combination with breathing techniques. Power yoga is a high-intensity yoga, popular in gyms, which focuses on flow from one pose to another and is primarily intended to build strength and flexibility. Iyengar, Anusara and Viniyoga are other common styles of yoga that are slow-paced and focus on alignment. Kripalu yoga is a slow-movement style that emphasizes mind/body awareness. Kundalini yoga uses more meditation, chanting and breathing along with poses.

A challenging type of yoga now commonly practiced in the United States is Ashtanga yoga, which features constant movement and breathing techniques. Through the movement, heat is generated which is felt to be vital to yogic practice. Bikram© yoga is another such yoga. Bikram yoga features 26 fixed postures, each repeated twice and performed in a room with 40 percent humidity, heated to more than 104° Fahrenheit. Practitioners often excessively sweat as they complete the postures. These higher intensity yoga are recommended for those who do not have ac-

FIGURE 2

NUMEROUS TYPES OF YOGA

Yoga is a physical, mental, and spiritual discipline
with a broad variety of schools, practices, and goals

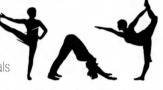

Style	Intensity	Highlights
▪ Hatha Yoga	Variable	Umbrella term for styles working with poses and breath
▪ Power Yoga	High	Continuous sequence of poses
▪ Iyengar/Anusara Yoga	Medium	Emphasis on proper alignment
▪ Kripalu Yoga	Low	Encourages mind/body awareness
▪ Kundalini Yoga	Low/Medium	Encourages self empowerment . utilizes chanting, poses and breath
▪ Ashtanga Yoga	High	Series of scripted poses-create your own heat focuses on rhythmic breathing
▪ Bikram Yoga	High	Series of scripted poses in artificial heat

tive medical issues. As you can see, there are many types of yoga, making it easy to individualize practice to fit each person's needs. *(Figure 2)*

We don't want people to get caught up in the type of yoga they practice because all types have health benefits. In clinical practice, yoga is prescribed to help with sleep problems; stress, balance or gait problems; and to assist with weight loss. Yoga can build muscle, improve memory and reduce pain.[278] [279] Done routinely, yoga arguably, comes closer than any other practice to a true "anti-aging" routine. The term "anti-aging," however, really is a misnomer. Goals of anti-aging are not to stop the aging process, but rather to age gracefully, which includes being disease-free and preserving vision, cognitive health and body structure. *(Consider 1)*

What good is living to one hun-

> # CONSIDER
>
> √ **What are our goals as we age?**
> Is it to fight the process of aging or is the goal really to age with grace and strength. We want to be disease free, have good vision, preserve memory and body structure. Yoga has been shown to help decrease chronic illness, preserve memory and maintain body structure.

dred years of age if you can't think clearly or perform your normal daily activities? The goal is to maintain a high quality of life as well as maintain independence. Yoga, as you will see, works on cognitive health, core strength and lowering inflammation, and limits the physical impacts of stress and hormone imbalance, which can be very effective for keeping cells from aging too quickly. It is accessible to everyone regardless of geographic location or socioeconomic class and can fit into any schedule. Once the basic techniques of yoga are learned, the goal should be to try to sustain a daily home practice.

In the West, yoga is often considered just another exercise. Although any yoga is helpful, the mindset of doing it at as an exercise once or twice a week neglects its potential health benefits. Traditionally, yoga is meant to be a daily practice, just like brushing your teeth or eating breakfast, though it can be done at any time. Perhaps the most simple yoga style is spending 15 minutes each day focusing on your breath while you move. This can be difficult in a world full of distractions that throw us out of balance all day long, but practicing yoga every day can help us. It can be difficult to calm the mind—but, like any exercise, this too takes practice.

A barrier for many is that yoga conjures up images of twisting the body into a pretzel, and the need to be highly flexible before you begin. We often hear, "I am not the yoga type," or, "My mind wanders too much. I have no patience for yoga." We started there, too. We used to be too impatient to hold a pose. We would get upset at our inflexibility and would count the seconds during a meditation. It is precisely those who lack flexibility, have poor balance, muscle weakness, and /or trouble focusing who benefit most from yoga. The key is persistence; once you learn from a knowledgeable practitioner who can teach you proper technique in the meditative, breathing and postural practices, you can begin a daily practice. We prefer in-person training at first so the teacher can correct alignment for poses, but internet videos, DVDs and CDs are great for learning breathing techniques and meditation.

Because yoga ideally combines breathing exercises, postures and meditation, many research studies focus on asanas (poses), pranayama (breathing exercises) and meditation together. The poses typically utilize isometric concepts. These build muscles by utilizing your body weight or holding a pose to cause muscle contraction and not bending at the joint as you would with free weights. The movement from one pose to another can be a terrific cardiovascular workout.

Pranayama breathing utilizes diaphragmatic (big belly) breathing and different speeds, durations and ratios of inhalations and exhalations. Our breath, especially exhaling, is a very powerful tool for activating our parasympathetic nervous system. When this occurs, our heart rate and breathing rate slow down. We are calmer. The parasympathetic, as you may recall, is our rest-and- recovery tool that balances our fight-or-flight component. *(Consider 2)*

Balance is essential. Most of us, again, push ahead on sympathetic overdrive and don't give enough focus to "rest and digest." Slow, methodical exhalations directly calm our nervous system by putting us into rest and recovery. Many of us have told someone who is very stressed (or been told ourselves), "Breathe!". It has been reported that the practice of pranayama modulates cardio-respiratory functions by increasing the input of the parasympathetic system.[280] Methodical breathing allows us to calm down our nervous system, slow our heart rate and has been shown to aid in digestive issues. One case study showed that heartburn was significantly improved in a man who followed a pranayama practice.[281] More studies are clearly needed to clarify the role yoga plays in GI issues. However, this particular study attributed the man's success to the increased tone of his diaphragm, which is a smooth muscle separating our abdominal and thoracic cavities. By strengthening this muscle, many believe less acid will travel from the stomach to the esophagus. *(Figure 3)*

> ## CONSIDER ❷
>
> √ **You always have one tool with you all of the time to calm down your stress response: your breathing rate and timing of inhalation and exhalation.** Try inhaling through your nose for a count of 4 and exhaling by mouth for a count of 8. Do this 5 times. Do you feel calmer?

THE MEDITATION ASPECT OF YOGA.

THE MEDITATION ASPECT OF YOGA is beneficial because it retrains the mind to create a calmer state. Then we can experience life without getting bogged down by anxiety and dread from fear of the unknown, uncertain futures or reliving past events. People who meditate can select from several techniques: some examples are focused attention, mindfulness and compassion meditation. Focused attention allows for a concentration on breath cycles, sound or chants; its goal is to train the mind from wandering and focus on a fixed task such as breathing.

Focusing on our breathing allows for fleeting thoughts to extinguish. Mindfulness is paying attention to the current moment's experience such as attention to breath, sounds, and thoughts but observing them and reacting without emotion. Guided meditation, which is where someone provides instructions during the meditation, is a form of mindfulness. Many have found that this form of meditation is a nice place to start a meditative practice. Guided meditation practice offers us exercises to train our minds to be mindful and allow us to be more in the moment. Compassion meditation cultivates feelings of benevolence towards other people.[282] It often employs a repetitive phrase to foster feelings of universal good, and is intended to decrease anxiety and burnout—especially useful for caregivers. *(Case 3)*

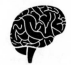

FIGURE 3

THE BENEFITS OF YOGA
positive effects on your mind and body

DECREASES	INCREASES
· Stress	· DHEA Hormone
· Inflammation	· Growth Hormone
· Cortisol	**IMPROVES**
· Fatigue	· Mood
· Weight	· Muscle Mass
· Blood Pressure	· Endothelial Function
· Mortality	· Cholesterol
· Rate of Heart Attacks	· Heart Rate
· Insulin Resistance	· Breathing Rate

These three techniques augment specific areas of the brain that relate to restfulness, but they also improve attention skills and reaction time to stimuli. These meditative techniques actually shrink areas of the brain involved with anxiety, rage and low mood. [283] In addition, the most exciting aspect of meditation for us is that meditation builds up the grey matter in the front of the brain=good thing. This is called the prefrontal cortex and is associated with working memory (or making new memories). A study from Harvard University showed that parts of the nerve cell called axons which transmits information to other cells can increase in the brain of those who meditate.[284] Other studies have shown that meditative practices like restful waking (lying awake in the dark and focusing on breathing) facilitate auditory learning.[285] This means that just the practice of resting and focusing on being calm can improve our ability to learn through hearing. Further, meditation can increase the connections between cells which will increase memory, overall brain function and resilience to stress.[286] In a time when the rates of Alzheimer's disease are exponentially increasing, this is very exciting information to potentially help us with the war against brain thinning (atrophy) and memory loss. *(Consider 3)*

Other roles for yoga, pranayama, and meditation are community geared. These goals are to create resiliency in residents of high risk areas, rehabilitation to those who have been imprisoned. Police Inspector Kiran Bedi used mindfulness breathing techniques to rehabilitate hardened criminals in Tihar Jail, one of the largest complexes of prisons in India. Her successful program educating the inmates about anger, fear and hatred and turning them into productive members of society, earned her international recognition and world praise.[287] Currently, programs are being instituted in select prisons from Seattle to DC in hopes of using it to reduce violence and crime.

Another example of the benefits of yoga in the community is seen with the Holistic Life Foundation[288] in Baltimore, Maryland. This foundation teaches meditation to teachers, parents and children. They began their work in areas of high risk such as inner-city Baltimore more than 10 years ago and have expanded to many other locations and demographic areas. The foundation offers residency programs where instructors teach mindfulness to children, helping them to cope with chronic stress and anxiety.

Other leaders such as Arianna Huffington, founder of Huffington Post, are trying to change the corporate culture by suggesting they add a daily meditation practice in the workplace, starting at the CEO

> ## Case 3
>
> **Dr R.: I used to see 25 people per day. Half way during the day, I was completely wiped out trying to give my patients full attention and empathy.** I would have to force myself to take 20 minutes and meditate. I would come back feeling recharged and ready to the rest of the day. It has always amazed me how relaxing the mind can recharge the whole body.

> ## CONSIDER
>
> √ Yoga is another tool which will help your memory, your ability to combat stress, and improve overall brain function.

level. Hopefully this cultural mindset of working and feeling guilty about taking time to recharge ourselves with tools like meditation will diminish when we see how productive and pleasant the workplace can be when people are recharged.

THE MULTI-TASKING ELEPHANT IN THE ROOM: Are we overdoing it?

ONE COMMON REAL-LIFE OCCURRENCE is how often Monica cannot find her car, when she returns to a parking lot after an errand. She is usually the one pressing her key alarm and listening for the sound of where her car is. Most of the time when she enters a building from a parking lot, she is catching up on phone calls, emails or texts and reviewing her overscheduled day. Does this sound familiar? Being more present at the task at hand would solve the problem. We often think such "forgetfulness" is a memory issue, but that is not completely true. Memory is not the problem. It is our lack of mindfulness – focusing on the moment and being present in the moment without letting distractions get in the way of the current moment.

Technology has changed our lives. The advent of smartphones, tablets and devices helps get us information quickly and stay connected to one another. We have a wealth of guidance at our fingertips. However, these high-tech toys also serve as a distraction and cause us to be less mindful. The constant buzz of incoming texts and social media messages takes us away from our thoughts and tasks. Multitasking is a misnomer and suggests efficiency; a better label would be, "rapid toggling between tasks."

> ## CONSIDER ❹
> **Have you noticed how often your phone "dings" during the day or during an hour?** In response, how often do you stop what you are doing to check the message. Consider how disruptive that is to your focus.

Bob Sullivan and Hugh Thompson, in their New York Times article "Brain, Interrupted," describe research done at Carnegie Mellon by Professor Acuisti.[289] The professor showed that an increase in interruptions results in 20 percent lower test scores. That multi-tasking and constant toggling between tasks worsens performance. We think we are being more efficient, but in the long run, our efficiency is less, and we actually perform worse. It's also important to incorporate technology-free times into your day so you can focus on family, relationships and calming the mind. *(Consider 4)*

YOGIC MINDFULNESS AND CHRONIC ILLNESS/LIFESPAN.

THE AVERAGE LIFESPAN around the world is increasing. The Centers for Disease Control (CDC) reports that life expectancy in the U.S. is at a record high of 78.8 years for those born in 2012 – females live for an average of 81.2 years and males live 76.4 years. As we age, the likelihood of contracting a chronic illness increases. With chronic illness, inflammation grows. We desperately need tools to help us age gracefully, preserve our mind and body structure, and improve our quality of life. One recent study linked loneliness in older adults to inflammation and showed that a mindfulness program reduces both inflammatory markers in the blood and feelings of loneliness.[290] *(Consider 5)*

> **CONSIDER ⑤**
>
> √ Consider that here is another tool to decrease the inflammation in our blood!

The goal of aging gracefully is to not live in a bubble. We cannot escape stress. It is part of life. But we can change the way in which our body perceives stress. Stress can be good because it raises our awareness. But it can also raise stress levels to a point where it causes anxiety and sleep disorders. Activation of sympathetic nervous system during the "alarm phase" or acute stress, can set up a cycle of high adrenaline leading to higher levels of cortisol which when left unchecked can cause the multiple symptoms of stress and lead to chronic illness. However, most forms of yoga recharge us and lower the cortisol surges.[291] [292] [293]

One study looked at women breast cancer survivors who had between stage II and stage IV breast cancers. Researchers found that regular yoga practice of 90 minutes, twice weekly for eight weeks, resulted in lower levels of both morning cortisol and evening cortisol levels and better overall well-being and fatigue scores.[294] These cancer patients felt better when they did yoga and their stress markers went down!

It is also worth noting that the aging person is not the only one who suffers when her health is poor. The caregivers who have the burden of providing care to the chronically ill also experience high levels of stress. Recall that stress triggers inflammation.[295] One study looked at the inflammatory markers of family members caring for parents with dementia. They found that those caregivers who meditated 12 minutes daily for eight weeks were able to decrease the inflammatory markers in their body. As people are living longer, there are many families providing care to the elderly. This finding reminds us that meditation is a great tool in calming stress and inflammation in this caregiver population.[296]

HORMONE IMBALANCE.

ONE OF THE MOST FRUSTRATING aspects of aging for both patients and physicians is hormone imbalance. Yoga has the ability to affect our hormone balance and speak directly to that stress response. More on this in a minute. First, let's talk about a few basics. Hormones are proteins in the body that communicate between different organs and tissues. They regulate most functions in the body such as (but not limited to) digestion, metabolism, sleep, reproduction and mood. Hormone imbalance and decline in most hormones are key factors in aging.

For example, Dehydroepiandrosterone (DHEA) and Growth hormone are naturally occurring hormones that decline as we age. DHEA has been linked to muscle mass, vitality and cognitive health. Growth hormone, which is secreted from the pituitary gland of the brain, is linked to our ability to grow and heal. One study looked at effects of regular yoga training for 12 weeks. Researchers observed that subjects who practiced yoga (using postures, breathing and meditation) had higher levels of DHEA and growth hormone. The training utilized breathing practices, mediation techniques, and poses in various combinations over different time durations.[297] Yoga is an amazing way to naturally elevate hormones, especially as we age.

Adiponectin is a hormone generated by fat tissue. It is key to the metabolism of fat and glucose. Visceral fat, or "belly fat," surrounds our internal organs. Excessive visceral fat is linked to an increase in inflammatory markers. Studies show yoga helps to reduce weight, improve muscle mass, decrease blood pressure, along with reducing inflammatory markers. Yoga also increases adiponectin levels, which then regulates glucose and fat metabolism and assists with weight management.[298] *(Figure 3)*

Other studies find yoga helps to reduce hormones associated with polycystic ovary syndrome (PCOS). PCOS is a disorder where the balance between a woman's estrogen and testosterone becomes imbalanced. Women will have excess testosterone leading to irregular menstrual cycles, acne, excessive hair growth, insulin resistance and infertility. Yoga has been shown to favorably impact glucose metabolism, lipids and hormone balance with PCOS. One study showed yoga was superior to exercise in lowering insulin resistance, which is a precursor to diabetes.[299]

CARDIOVASCULAR BENEFITS.

S TRESS IS INCREASINGLY IDENTIFIED as a culprit in cardiovascular illness. The link is felt to be through the effects of cortisol and the sympathetic nervous system.[300] Stress appears to trigger endothelial dysfunction (inability of the blood vessels to dilate appropriately). Damage to the endothelium has been implicated in the formation of plaque. One study looked at healthy men who were given a mental stress test; researchers found that after periods of mental stress, the healthy men had endothelial dysfunction for up to four hours.[301] It is amazing to think that our stress can trigger heart disease. This further emphasizes the importance of having tools to decrease stress.

In another study, stress reduction techniques such as yoga and meditation were examined in 33 people with and without heart disease. Participants meditated and did yoga for weeks. In the patients with cardiovascular disease, yoga and meditation improved endothelial function significantly.[302] Although this particular study did not find significant change in endothelial function in the non-heart disease patients, they did find a decrease in blood pressure, heart rate and BMI (body mass index) in both the patients with and without heart disease.

Even with all of our current advances in knowledge, medications, procedures and surgical interventions, cardiovascular disease still remains the leading cause of death in Americans. Pioneers in lifestyle medicine like Dr. Dean Ornish realized more than 30 years ago that lifestyle changes, including stress reduction strategies such as yoga and meditation combined with dietary changes, can reduce risk factors for cardiac health. With these lifestyle changes, parameters that improved were cholesterol, endurance, work performance and heart function.[303]More recently, the European Journal of Clinical Cardiology looked at more than 37 randomized controlled trials on asana based yoga practice, and found lower cardiovascular risk factors such as BMI, systolic blood pressure, lower total cholesterol, triglyceride and LDL levels. Higher HDL levels were also noted. They concluded that there is promising evidence for yoga's improving heart health.[304] In fact, when comparing participants who did yoga but no traditional cardiovascular exercise to those who did traditional exercise, the study showed there was no difference in their heart health. It suggests that yoga shows promise in improving cardiovascular health.

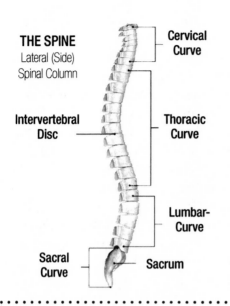

THE SPINE
Lateral (Side)
Spinal Column

Cervical
Curve

Intervertebral
Disc

Thoracic
Curve

Lumbar-
Curve

Sacral
Curve

Sacrum

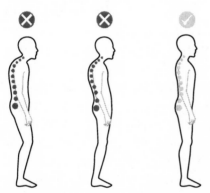

Incorrect Versus Correct Standing Posture

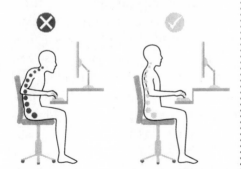

Incorrect Versus Correct Sitting Posture

Figure 4
Your Spine:
Posture & Alignment

With good posture and a neutral spine, we have a slight cervical curve (anteriorly or towards the front of the body), thoracic curvature posteriorly, and lumbar curvature anteriorly. **Sitting at a desk causes forward protrusion of the neck,** which can result in not only cervical or neck issues but also upper back and shoulder issues due to the trapezius muscle that connects them.

YOGA AND MOOD.

MOOD ISSUEs are another area in which we as clinicians like to give patients lifestyle tools. One mindfulness program initiated by Dr. Jon Kabat-Zinn at the University of Massachusetts, entitled Mindfulness Based Stress Reduction (MBSR) has become quite popular. He has created an eight week program that teaches mindfulness in a stepwise fashion. Kabat-Zinn's programs have been studied in trial and have been found to deliver significant benefits so that more than 250 hospitals worldwide use it as an adjunct to health care in a variety of areas.

MBSR has been used successfully in Irritable Bowel

Syndrome patients which has a significant stress component. There has always been a strong connection between mood and the gut. IBS is considered a functional illness because its symptoms, such as bloating, gas, constipation alternating with diarrhea, relate to the gut's functions, but there are no structural, infectious or microscopic changes in the gut. Often, these symptoms are triggered by emotion. It is a very common diagnosis with limited treatment options, which frustrates both patients and providers. However, in one study, the group who completed the MBSR training showed a reduction in the severity of symptoms of IBS and the symptoms of stress which were maintained at the 6 month follow up.[305] One of the most exciting studies recently published was conducted at Johns Hopkins University in March, 2014. This study reviewed more than 18,000 meditation studies over 47 different trials and found that mindfulness programs improved levels of anxiety, depression and pain. [306]

In areas where stress can play a large role in flares, such as with inflammatory bowel disease, research has showed that those patients with the highest stress markers (measured by urinary cortisol) were the ones who reported better quality of life scores with mindfulness, even during their flares.[307] If we extrapolate from this, then mindfulness will have benefit in so many chronic illness.

YOGA NIDHRA.

OUR FAVORITE TYPE OF YOGA is called yoga nidhra, which allows us to enter a state between wakefulness and sleep.[308] Yoga nidhra is referred to as yogic sleep and is a practice in which you lie in sivasana (corpse pose) and utilize breathing techniques, followed by periods of focusing on one body part at a time, then follow a guided meditation. It has been show to induce an alpha wave brain wave state which is associated with a relaxed mental state. Yoga nidhra improves in restful sleep but does not have to be done at night. It recharges the autonomic nervous system by improving the parasympathetic (rest and digest) component. It is an excellent tool for facilitating sleep when a person is aroused at night. (Consider 6)

> **CONSIDER** ⑥
>
> √ Do you find that you have difficulty calming your racing mind when you wake up at night? Yoga nidhra can be a great tool for this.

TRANSCENDENTAL MEDITATION.

TRANSCENDENTAL MEDITATION (TM) is another specific form of mind/body intervention that has generated compelling data regarding cardiovascular medicine. It is a form of meditation that uses a mantra—a word or sound which has phonetic significance in order to settle the mind. TM is a technique performed for 20 minutes, twice a day. Some benefits have related to a drop in cortisol levels of up to 30 percent.[309] [310] Studies show that a TM practice reduces sympathetic nervous system activation.[311] These findings of lower cortisol and decreased sympathetic activation have shown benefit in areas such as cardiovascular disease. One study showed that TM reduced the risk of mortality, myocardial infarction (MI) and stroke in patients with a history of heart disease.[312] In fact, the American Heart Association recommends the use of TM for prevention and treatment of hypertension.[313]

ALIGNMENT

YOGA ALSO INCORPORATES A FOCUS on posture and alignment. Poor posture and alignment have been linked to many medical disorders. A curved spine as a result of sitting for 8 to10 hours per day has many detrimental effects, not only on our stature but it also can be the source of pain issues, decreased energy and play a role in other chronic disease states. Regarding chronic illness, prolonged sitting can cause our muscles to utilize insulin less effectively. This can directly lead to issues with glucose metabolism and eventually with insulin resistance and pre-diabetes. Prolonged sitting can also be associated with pain syndromes. Strained neck, carpal tunnel, shoulder pain and lower back and hip pain can all arise from sitting. In an age when most us sit, —commute to work and sit in a car for two hours per day and then sit at a desk for eight hours, our posture and alignment suffer.

Normal alignment requires three curves of the spine, which contain 33 bones arranged as cervical (C1-C7), thoracic (T1-T12), lumbar (L1-L5) and sacral (S1-S5). *(Figure 4)*. With good posture and a neutral spine, we have a slight cervical curve (anteriorly or towards the front of the body), thoracic curvature posteriorly, and lumbar curvature anteriorly. Sitting at a desk at work and typing can all put a large strain on many different parts of this system. For instance, sitting at a desk causes forward protrusion of the neck, which can result in not only cervical or neck issues but also upper back and shoulder issues. The counter balance is to keep the shoulder relaxed, keep the neck from not leaning forward, sitting with the pelvic muscles flexed and keeping the feet flat on the floor.

Sitting for long periods also causes tightening of the hip flexors and weakness in the gluteal and abdominal muscles. This can lead to stiffness, inflexibility and can impact our discs. It also causes instability and increases our risk of falling. Yoga poses can combat these issues by its focus on lateral movement, extension of spine and balance. Imagine how good you feel when you do a light stretch after prolonged sitting; now imagine what a daily practice with yoga can do for combating the stress on our bodies from our daily routines.

Diaphragmatic breathing, which is a form of breathing in yoga, can utilize shoulder, thorax and abdominal muscles more efficiently if done periodically during the work day. In fact, one study meta-analysis showed an improvement in lung flow for patients with chronic obstructive pulmonary disease (COPD) when practicing yoga.[314] The mechanism is not clear, but it may involve relaxing the body as well as improved muscle function. It also allows for a focus on neutral alignment, which benefits air entry.

Many yoga poses, such as downward facing dog or the cat and cow pose, work on the opposing muscles which are contracted while sitting all day. Adding stretches and yoga poses into your day or using a sit-stand desk can help protect against adverse health effects caused by sitting eight hours a day. There are many websites available that summarize up-to-date research on the benefits of sit/stand desks.

Expert opinion and research has shown that prolonged sitting can have an effect on our response to insulin. The Washington Post ran an article in January, 2014, showing the hazards of sitting on many organs in the body. The authors showed a decrease in appropriate insulin response after only one day of prolonged sitting.[315] Other studies show that yoga postures and meditation reduce fasting glucose and insulin levels, suggesting that the pancreas becomes more sensitive to glucose signals and does not have to work as hard. We can now consider using yoga to decrease our sugar levels.[316] [317]

PELVIC FLOOR.

WOMEN OFTEN EXPERIENCE DIFFICULTY with holding their urine at one time or another. This is called stress incontinence and can often be triggered by excessive impact as with running, excess weight and multiple pregnancies. Stress incontinence can also happen with hormone changes in menopause. Symptoms are frustrating to women who often have to urinate frequently and have small amounts of urine "leakage" when coughing, sneezing, laughing or exercising. Pelvic floor yoga (yoga which works on the muscles and ligaments and nerves that support organs such as bladder, uterus, rectum and vagina) is a great tool for combating urinary incontinence. Our pelvic floor muscles are "use-it-or-lose-it" muscles. We need to work on them actively to maintain them. Kegel exercises are a type of pelvic floor exercise that utilizes contractions of the pelvic floor muscles for 5 to 10 seconds to mimic the cessation of urine flow. These work but they need to be done several times each day. We recommend linking Kegel exercises to an activity that happens often in your day, such as receiving a phone call or sending an email. However, adding pelvic floor yoga takes it to a new level. We have found pregnancy yoga tapes to be helpful for bladder strengthening. These exercises are simple and can be done sitting in a chair even when at work.

DOES YOGA AFFECT OUR GENES TOO?

WE FEEL THAT THE MOST IMPACTFUL ASPECT OF YOGA is the effect on our genes, the parts of the parts of the body which determine who we are. Many people believe that their genes control their destiny. In fact, very few genetic disorders are fixed. Most genetic predispositions are affected by the environment. Lifestyle factors such as activity, food choices and environmental insults such as viral exposure and toxins can change the way our genes manifest. Studies now show that yoga directly affects the way our genes are expressed. [318]

There are also studies showing that relaxation responses such as yoga, meditation and breathing can enhance the energy powerhouse of cells called mitochondria, by impacting the genes that regulate the energy producing reactions of our body.[319] Energy is created is through formation of ATP (adenosine triphosphate). Relaxation response has been shown to increase ATP and therefore, increases mitochondrial energy production. This makes us more effective at utilizing our supply and balancing with demand. At the same time, these practices have been shown to decrease inflammation causing decreasing production of proteins (such as NF-KB) which turn on inflammation cascades in the body. Lower levels of NF-KB in immune cells have also been correlated with lower oxidative stress. These data suggest that yoga can positively affect our energy, inflammation and oxidative stress pathways which are all implicated in chronic disease and aging.

Yoga is the ultimate way to combat many negative aspects of aging. In addition to genetic influence, it works on hormone imbalance, structural imbalance and inflammation, reduction in muscle mass, sleep disorders, poor cognitive health and mood disorders. Yoga's flexibility with utilizing meditation, breathing techniques and postures has a way of improving quality of life even when a patient suffers from chronic medical illness. Yoga, quite simply, is the ultimate anti-aging tool! The most beneficial aspects of yoga are the focus on Sivasana or concept of complete rest; the asanas that work on resistance, balance and stretching; and pranayama which allows us to be mindful and work on diaphragmatic breathing. Remember, yoga helps control cortisol and directly stimulates the parasympathetic nervous system, which combats many of the imbalances causing chronic disease.

For *Case 2* from the beginning of the chapter, Dr. Rao did recommend he try to practice mindfulness—do things with a focus on the current task, and don't get sidetracked by cell phone calls or texts while he is working on a specific task. Plan for technology-free time, focus on getting restorative sleep with yoga nidhra and practice meditation at least five times a week. That could mean doing anything mindfully – staring at a candle for five minutes, ironing, swimming or a yoga class. In the end, it does not matter which type it is; it's how often you do it that counts. Make mindfulness a daily practice. Just take a deep diaphragmatic breath and swan dive into it! *

YOUR PRESCRIPTION:

❶ Whatever method of yoga or meditation you decide to do, do it everyday

❷ Learn deep breathing techniques

❸ Make technology-free time everyday

❸ Focus on each task individually and avoid multitasking

CHAPTER 14:

The Euphoria of Exercise

Movement to reverse the damage
of a sedentary lifestyle

ONE OF DR. RAO'S PATIENTS IS A 36-YEAR-OLD WOMAN, *who came to the office with symptoms of excessive sweating. The symptoms started more than three month prior and she would sweat all over her body and at inappropriate times. She also had been experiencing significant diarrhea. She had been treated for depression in the past, and had been taking an anti-depressant called Duloxetine. She denied any change in her stress level or in the dose of her medication. Otherwise she had been feeling well in terms of energy and stamina. In fact, she reported she had been exercising more and was training for a half-marathon. Her symptoms worried her and she wanted to rule out cancer.*

Her initial testing and chest x-ray were all normal. Dr. Rao thought that perhaps her medication was creating side effects. This possibility surprised the patient as she had been taking the Duloxetine for five years; she couldn't understand why it suddenly could have an adverse effect after taking it consistently for so long. Dr. Rao believed that her recent exercise surge was raising the levels of neurotransmitters (chemical "messengers" in the brain that are responsible for good mood). As a result, her dose had become too high for her. While she felt a good deal of anxiety about this possibility, the patient ultimately agreed to taper the dose, and her symptoms resolved without any rebound in her depression. As it turned out, her high dose of Duloxetine was competing with the natural effects of running. Her sweating and other symptoms improved significantly after Dr. Rao cut the amount of antidepressant she took daily. She continued to run and felt great.

Exercise is defined as any physical activity done for a certain purpose. It is a regular, repeated activity that improves our physical fitness. For centuries, wellness advocates have promoted exercise as a way to boost health and avoid chronic illness. People who exercise can feel their heart rates increase, their muscles get stronger, and their speed increase. They have more power, agility, balance and coordination.

But those "body improvements" aren't the only reasons to exercise. Deliberate movement also improves our reaction time. We sweat, which drives out toxins from our bodies. Exercise also creates a feeling of euphoria and a sense of happiness; it gives us added energy,[320] improves our quality of life [321]and our ability to think more clearly. [322]

Physiologic parameters also improve with exercise. We see improvements in endurance, strength, flexibility and better body composition (muscle /fat ratios). Exercise brings healthy changes to blood sugar levels, cholesterol and metabolism. It lowers our risk of heart disease, stroke, type 2 diabetes, and certain types of cancers such as breast and colon. Studies have even shown that death from all causes (all-cause mortality) can be delayed by regular physical activity.[323]

HOW MUCH EXERCISE THE "RIGHT" AMOUNT?

IN 2007, THE AMERICAN HEART ASSOCIATION and The American College of Sports Medicine released guidelines to help both physicians and patients decide which activities people should undertake, and how much they should do each week, in order to achieve their goals. Recommendations for overall activity will be discussed in this chapter, but specific advice for goals such as weight loss, faster speed or athletic performance, or cardiovascular retraining should be personalized with the help of a physician. Generally speaking, the American Heart Association recommends 150 minutes of at least moderate exercise per week which can be broken down into 30-60 minutes sessions, five days per week. The guidelines recommend increasing intensity and frequency over time for maximum benefit. [324]

We often measure exercise intensity by the concept of Metabolic Equivalents of Task (MET) per week. A MET is a measure of energy expenditure of a physical activity. It is used to gauge the intensity of that activity. As we exercise, we need more air so we can get oxygen into our bloodstream and into our muscles. METs represent the oxygen uptake required relative to rest. For example, 6 METS means the oxygen required is six times that needed when at rest. One MET is what occurs

Figure 1
Metabolic Equivalents of Task
Measure of Energy Expenditure of a Physical Activity.

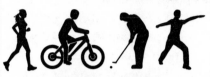 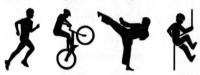

| MODERATE ACTIVITY 3.0 to 6.0 METs* | VIGOROUS ACTIVITY Greater than 6.0 METs* |

MODERATE ACTIVITY
3.0 to 6.0 METs*

WALKING *at a moderate or brisk pace of 3 to 4.5 mph on a level surface inside or outside, such as*

- Walking to class, work, or the store
- Walking for pleasure
- Walking the dog
- Walking as a break from work
- Walking downstairs or down a hill

GENERAL HOME EXERCISES
Light or moderate effort

* **Getting up and down** from the floor
* **Trampoline Jumping**
* **Stair Climber**
* **Rowing Machine**

ACTIVITIES MODERATE

* **Bicycling 5-9 mph**, level terrain, few hills
* **Stationary Bicycling**—moderate effort
* **Racewalking**—*less than 5 mph*
* **Hiking**
* **Roller skating**
* **Aerobic Dancing**—high impact
* **Water Aerobics**

SPORTS MODERATE

* **Golf** — walking with caddy
* **Tennis (doubles)**
* **Badminton**

VIGOROUS ACTIVITY
Greater than 6.0 METs*

WALKING, JOGGING

* **Race and aerobic walking**—5 mph
* **Jogging or running**
* **Wheeling your wheelchair**
* **Walking and climbing briskly up a hill**
* **Backpacking**

BICYCLING

* **Bicycling** more than 10 mph or uphill
* **Stationary Bicycling**—vigorous effort

EXERCISES VIGOROUS

* **Calisthenics**—push-ups, pull-ups,
* **Jumping Jacks**
* **Water Jogging**
* **Stair Climber Machine**—fast pace
* **Rowing Machine**
* **Arm Cycling Machine**

ACTIVITIES VIGOROUS

* **Roller Skating**—brisk pace
* **Aerobics: Step and Dancing**
* **Karate, judo, tae kwon do, jujitsu**
* **Mountain Rock Climbing, Rappelling**

SPORTS VIGOROUS

* **Tennis**
* **Basketball**
* **Swimming Laps**
* **Surf Boarding**

when quietly sitting and 3 METs is equal to three times the energy of sitting. Twenty-three METs is equivalent to running a mile in 4.17 minutes. METs are calculated in a sample population. METs are based on the average person but vary based on age and conditioning. For instance, a person who is 40 years old and has a high fitness level can walk at a pace of 3 to 4mph which is equal to 3 METs for him but for a 70-year-old man, that level would be considered more vigorous exercise and is closer to 6-7 METS. METs give us general guidelines to assess a person's exercise capacity. Overall, moderate intensity exercise is considered exercise that results in 3-6 METs. Examples of such exercise are walking at a brisk pace for 3-4.5 mph, hiking, roller skating, cycling at 5-9 mph, water aerobics and carrying your clubs with golf. The chart on the prior page can serve as a reasonable guideline.[325] *(Figure 1)*

Population studies looking at both men and women have showed that when they exercised at a workload of 3-5.9 METs (moderate activity) for 150 minutes per week, there was a significantly decreased risk of heart disease and mortality.[326] [327] [328] [329] [330] Further studies show that when a sedentary lifestyle is broken up by bursts of activity, the risk of chronic illness is attenuated.[331]

Ultimately, we know that all movement is important. Often people when told to exercise imagine that we are telling them to go for a five mile run. Exercise is all active movement. Movement can be active gardening, playing tennis or going for a walk. It can be yoga, jumping through the waves at the beach or canoeing. There are so many ways to be active. We just need to do something every day.

CURRENT STATE OF AFFAIRS: THE COACH POTATO

THESE STANDARDS WRITTEN by the American Heart Association and American College of Sports Medicine have been supported by numerous trials. The problem is that as a society, we have had trouble following them. Overall, we are a fairly sedentary society. We sit behind our desks for eight hours a day, sit in our cars with long commute times, and watch TV or sit in front of the computer in the evenings before bed. People often say they don't have time or are too tired to exercise after a long day at work.

With our sedentary lifestyle, obesity rates have risen: America's Health Rankings, a study by the American Public Health Association, reported in December 2014[332] that 29.4 percent of us are obese. It also highlighted that up to 23.5% of Americans are sedentary or reported no physical activity in the 30 days preceding the report. Research shows that a sedentary lifestyle directly increases risk of coronary heart disease, depression,[334] increases waist circumference, elevates blood pressure, worsens our lipid profiles[335], and increases biomarkers such as glucose and insulin (i.e. precursors to diabetes).

While a sedentary life can increase our risk of chronic illness, we also know that small increases in physical activity can then reduce our risk of heart disease, stroke, type 2 diabetes, and certain cancers. [336] Small increases in movement can reduce mortality from all causes by 20-30%. [337] That means that any amount of exercise will make you live longer. Small changes such as taking walking breaks during work, doing regular stretches or increasing steps per day even by 2,000 steps can help reduce our risk of serious illness. [338 339] In one study, when sedentary people started walking 10,000 steps per day for three days a week, their cholesterol levels plummeted.[340] Walking an additional 2,000 steps per day was associated with a decrease in systolic blood pressure by 4mmHg.[341 342]

As we become more active, however, we need to move more to achieve benefit. The minimum at that point is not enough. Exercise has to reach a certain level of intensity, which is unique to each individual's fitness level and health status. If the exercise does not tax the body enough, the changes won't be as noticeable.

Of note, there is a phenomenon termed the "active coach potato." That term applies to the many of us out there who satisfy the 150 minutes of moderate exercise per week but then the remainder of the time, we sit. Unfortunately, there is data coming out to suggest that even though we exercise, it is not okay then to be sedentary the remaining time and that there are metabolic consequences to this behavior.[343] The studies were done on people who were spending excessive time watching television but would apply to anyone who sits at a desk job

CONSIDER

Even though we cannot change our work or commute times, there are things we can change.

√ Take the stairs instead of the elevator at work

√ Park further away from the entrance to work

√ Decrease screen time

√ Go for a walk during lunch

and has long commuting times. Changes such as a sit/stand desk and activity during the day at work are of significant benefit. Think about the walk at lunch break, climbing stairs instead of using the elevator and walking to and from work. We also have to minimize our screen time in the evenings to combat our "couch potato" persona. Consider cutting back on television, computer and tablet time at the end of the day and go for a nice evening walk. *(Consider 1)*

EXERCISE DOES NOT ALWAYS EQUAL WEIGHT LOSS.

THE AMERICAN COLLEGE OF SPORTS MEDICINE recommends a range of 150 to 400 kcal of energy expenditure per day. A Kcal is short for kilocalorie and is a unit of energy. It can be used to quantitate how much energy from food you take in or how much energy you burn. Often calorie is interchanged with kilocalorie as an equivalent. The amount of calories a person will lose is highly variable. Calories burned depend on your body habitus (height, weight) as well as the length and intensity of the exercise. For instance, with a 160 pound man, one hour of cycling burns about 292 calories. One hour of water aerobics burns 402 calories for the same size person. Golf and carrying clubs burns 314 calories. [344] However, if a person is double that weight, the same activity will cause a significantly higher calorie loss. The larger you are, the more effort is required to move and therefore, more calories are lost. For example a 160 pound person walking at a pace of 3.5 miles

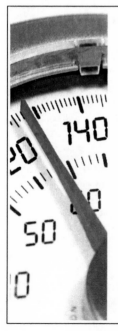

Figure 2:
CALORIES BURNED
based on body weight and activity of one hour duration
Adapted from the mayoclinic.org

Physical Activity	160 LB PERSON Calories Burned	240 LB PERSON Calories Burned
Running 5mph	606	905
High Impact Aerobics	533	796
Swimming Laps moderate	423	632
Water Aerobics	402	600
Low Impact Aerobics	365	545
Elliptical Trainer moderate effort	365	545
Golf with carrying clubs	314	469
Walking 2mph	204	305

per hour (mph) can burn 314 calories in an hour where as someone who weighs 240lbs, burns 469 calories for that same hour.[345] *(Figure 2)*

Not all exercise will cause weight loss, however. Weight loss is based on so many factors: how much we intake, how much we sleep, our hormone balance. Weight loss to some extent is dictated by supply versus demand. In order to lose weight, the amount we intake must be less than what we lose through movement. Often, after initial quick weight loss, people often plateau. Our bodies need more intensity of exercise then to increase the calorie burn rate. Sometimes it is as easy as walking for an extra ten minutes or adding weights while you walk. It is amazing how these small changes make huge differences.

WHAT IS EXERCISE ON A BIOCHEMISTRY LEVEL?

WHEN WE LOOK AT EXERCISE, we see it in terms of metabolic fitness, which is what happens to the body on a cellular and hormonal level. Metabolic fitness can be divided into aerobic (with oxygen) and anaerobic (without oxygen). Both cause our heart rate to increase and but have a very different role in our health.

Exercise creates a physical stress in which your body demands more oxygen, blood flow and nutrients, and energy production in muscles to sustain activity. More activity creates a greater demand for oxygen. When we exercise, our cells use a form of energy called ATP (adenosine triphosphate). During exercise, our bodies use glucose (sugar) and fat to make this energy so that we can keep going. We metabolize sugar or fat based on whether oxygen is present or not in our system.

At the beginning of an exercise session, we are primarily doing aerobic fitness because we have adequate oxygen to perform the required tasks at the beginning of our routines. Our heart rates increase to bring oxygenated blood to the muscles we are using. With oxygen, our bodies break down fat to make ATP so that our bodies can work more effectively. Although glucose is also being used in aerobic, the primary substrate is fat. For this reason, people often call aerobic fitness the "fat burn" stage of exercise. *(Figure 3)*

As we do more endurance work, our muscles demand oxygen and nutrients and our muscles run out of oxygen. We breathe faster to bring in more oxygen and our heart rates go up to get the oxygen to the muscles that need it. Over time, however, we cannot get enough oxygen to the muscles that require it. Our muscle cells then shift to working without oxygen (anaerobic metabolism). Without oxygen,

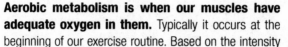

FIGURE 3

Aerobic versus Anaerobic Metabolism

Aerobic metabolism is when our muscles have adequate oxygen in them. Typically it occurs at the beginning of our exercise routine. Based on the intensity of our workout, aerobic metabolism can continue as long as our heart rates stay in the aerobic zone. As intensity and duration pick up, our muscles become depleted of oxygen and the body changes to anaerobic metabolism. It is then the muscles find other sources of energy, i.e. glucose. The byproduct of this metabolism is lactic acid which makes our muscles sore after workouts

AEROBIC EXERCISE	ANAEROBIC EXERCISES
• **Utilizes oxygen**	• **Without oxygen**
• **More efficient** –releases more energy	• **Less efficient**- releases less energy
• **Able to sustain for long periods**	• **More for high intensity**
• **Utilizes more fat** more than glucose	• **Utilizes glucose**
• **By products are CO2,** water and energy	• **Creates lactic acid** which can cause muscle fatigue
• **Works at heart rates** under 70% max HR	• **Works at heart rates over** 80% of max HR
• **Can talk through**	• **Unable to talk through** feels uncomfortable
• **Endurance workouts**	• **High intensity interval training,** strength training with weights

the body does not break down fat. It transitions to using glucose as the primary source of fuel for energy. When we use glucose without oxygen, lactic acid is the by-product. Lactic acid in our muscles is what makes them ache after a good workout. To help clear away the lactic acid, we activate our sympathetic nervous system (our fight or flight response) with the neurotransmitter norepinephrine (also called adrenaline). This allows our heart rate and blood pressure to further elevate and help bring more oxygen supply to our muscles.

This process of activating the nervous system is a form of stress. Exercise, though is initially a *eustress* because the increases in heart rate and blood pressure allow our supply to keep up with demand. The increase in heart rate also helps bring more oxygen to the tired muscles and aid in removing lactic acid. If we continue exercising, we accumulate even more lactic acid and speed up our heart rate even more. Eventually, based on our fitness levels, the muscles fatigue and we stop exercising.

Exercising beyond our fitness level becomes a *distress*. We become unbalanced and overwork our sympathetic nervous system. There is more adrenaline and the heart rate stays higher. Over time, this can cause injury and symptoms of overtraining, which can tax our immune systems.[346] Overdoing exercise will initially look like excessive muscle soreness and fatigue. With chronic imbalance, we start seeing difficulty sleeping, recurrent sicknesses/infections, mood disorders and immune dysregulation. The immune system doesn't work as well. This is why it's important to build up slowly to an optimal fitness level.

A key regulator for increased oxygen and nutrients to the muscle is dilation of the blood vessels. Blood flow to the muscles can increase 85% when we exercise compared to blood flow when we rest.[347] Dilating your blood vessels is key to sustained exercise because this gives the vessels the ability to open up and handle that giant increase in blood flow. This action creates a positive feedback look and enables the heart to pump more oxygenated blood to the body, then to the muscle.

Blood vessel dilation is brought about by a substance called nitric oxide (NO). The discovery of nitric oxide has been crucial to our understanding of disease states in general. For instance, in heart disease caused by high blood pressure, cholesterol, diabetes and other risk factors, our blood vessel linings can't produce adequate amounts of nitric oxide. As a result, the vessels are often small and unable to dilate and accommodate the change in blood flow required by the demands of movement and exercise. Recall, this is endothelial dysfunction. When blood flow in the heart arteries is restricted, the heart pump itself suffers, and our bodies feel chest pain or angina.

As physicians, we recommend increasing exercise capacity because we know the nitric oxide stores will build over time with continued exercise.[348] Exercise not only helps healthy blood vessels dilate but will ultimately help dilate the thin, restricted vessels – and, over time, the angina will diminish.[349] [350] Exercise, however, should be done with caution and only after consultation with your physician. Further, we know that increasing nitric oxide can help prevent platelet aggregation (or platelet clumping), thus reducing the rate of plaque formation in your arteries.[351]

Figure 4:

Sources Of Plant Based
Branched Chain Amino Acids

helpful after a workout to build new muscle

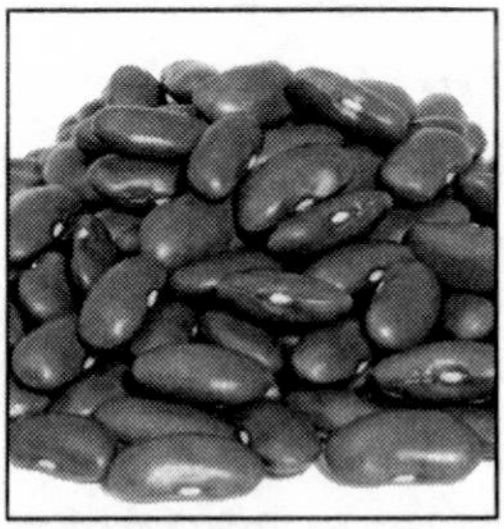

Beans	Lentils	Pumpkin seeds
Brazil nuts	Walnuts	Cashews

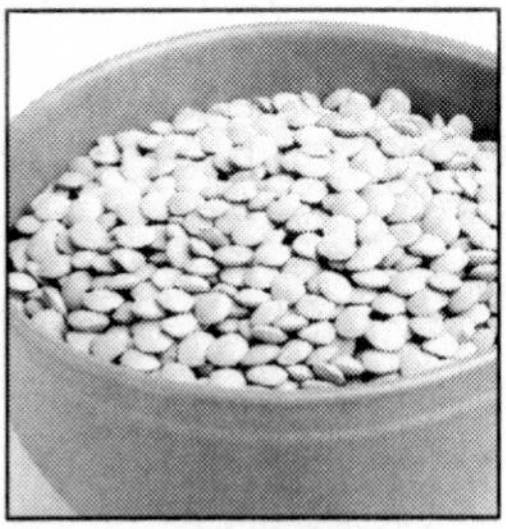

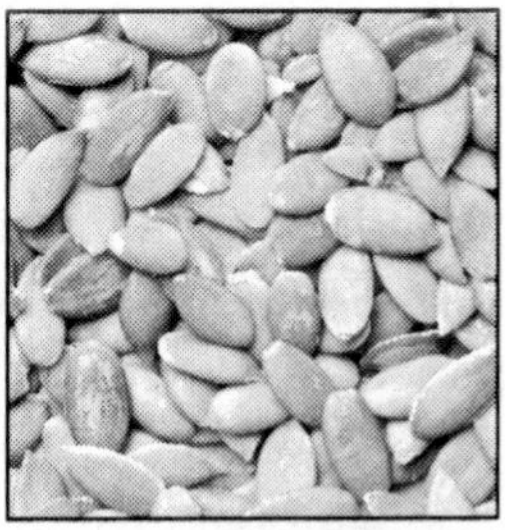

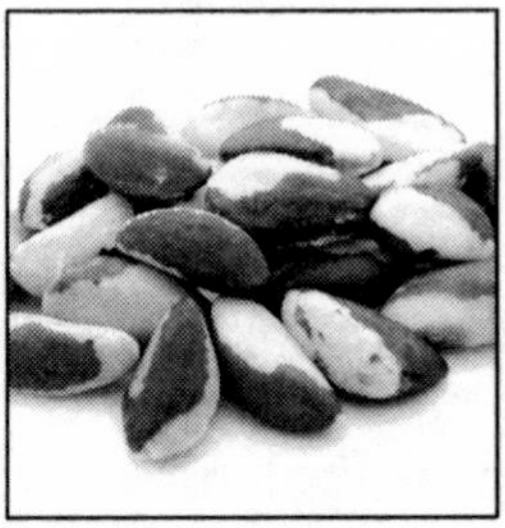

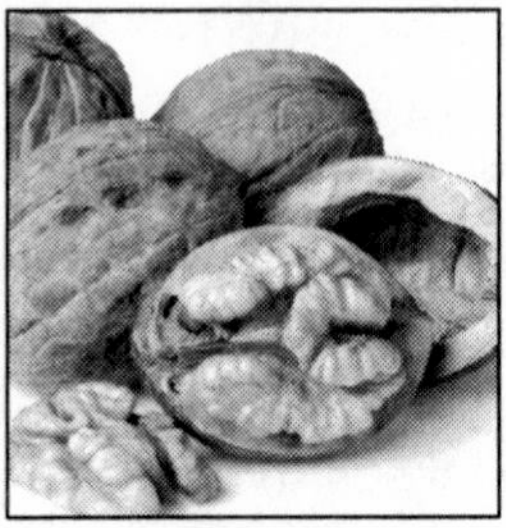

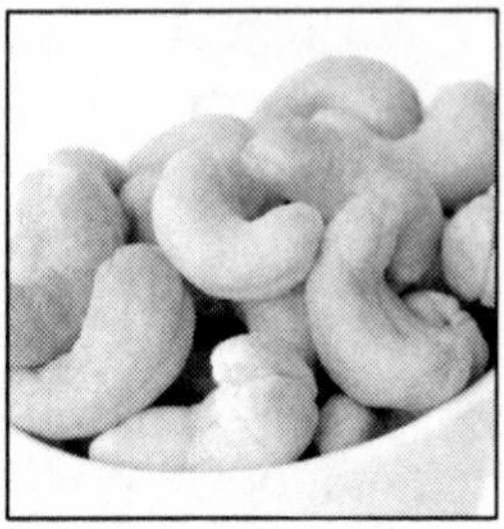

While blood flow to our muscles and heart increases when we exercise, it also increases blood flow to our skin, which helps dissipate the heat of muscle activity. However, because of this sympathetic overdrive, the blood vessels to the other nonessential organs constrict to conserve resources. That is why, if we eat and then exercise too soon, we cramp. The body has pulled its blood flow away from the stomach to focus on movement and will only be allowed to fully metabolize that food when the parasympathetic is activated and recovery begins. In general, it's advisable not to eat heavy foods up to one hour prior to exercise.

IT'S NOT ALL ABOUT THE WORKOUT: GIVING TIME TO REFUEL

POSITIVE STRUCTURAL and functional changes in our bodies occur with exercise and allow for our body to adapt to increased demands on the body. These adaptations occur during recovery. The body needs time to remove the waste from our cells, allow for the generation of new muscle and form the necessary factors for generating energy production.[352] There needs to be time between workouts to allow for this process to occur. Especially when first starting an exercise program, it is advisable to allow one day between workouts of similar muscle groups. For instance, if we go for a run one day, then the next day we should not run. We should swim or do a cross training/core exercise, or play tennis etc. Giving breaks between work outs allow for the body to build up nutrients for the next workout, and also to recover from the small injuries on a microscopic level that occur during exercise. Along with appropriate time between workouts, other factors such as balanced nutrition, proper hydration, avoidance of extreme temperature can affect recovery. There is some debate about the right amount of carbohydrates to protein ratio for workout before, during and after workouts but dietary intake needs to be tailored to the intensity and type of work outs. For example, intake of carbohydrates within 2 hours after a high endurance workout like a marathon is recommended to replace lost stores. Branched chain amino acids which are building blocks for protein are helpful after a workout to help build new muscle.[353] We can get these branch chain amino acids from beans, lentils, pumpkin seeds, brazil nuts, walnuts and cashews.[354] Remember, we need to take the time to restore balance with these changes after significant exercise. *(Figure 4)*

If this time and support is not allotted, fatigue and muscle soreness can set in. If the body continues to be stressed, performance can fall and you can develop an overreaching syndrome. The fatigue and muscle soreness with overreaching syndrome can last from two weeks to two months, depending on the severity. Additional symptoms can be insomnia, increased immune dysfunction, and the start of worsen-

FIGURE 5:

SPECTRUM OF EXERCISE LEADING TO OVERTRAINING

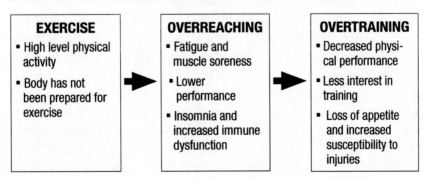

ing allergies. It is felt that we are susceptible to this imbalance because of lower glycogen stores, decreased branched chain amino acids, increased oxidative stress and increased stress on the hormone and immune system. Relative rest and support of nutrients and hydration usually resolve this issue.[355]

If we don't heal our overreaching syndrome,, we can worsen the imbalance and develop the syndrome of overtraining. Overtraining exhibits itself as decreased physical performance, less interest in training, elevated resting heart rate, and poor concentration. In overtraining, we also see mood alterations, loss of appetite and increased susceptibility to injuries. This can last from 8 weeks to 3 months even with rest. [356] Although rare, this spectrum of overreaching and overtraining syndrome is not just for the highly trained athlete, it can happen for those who do high level physical activity bursts where the body has not been prepared for the intensity of the exercise. In this situation, adaptation is markedly impaired and homeostasis is disturbed. This is why starting low and going slow with exercise is a good idea but taking adequate rest between sessions can help prevent these detrimental changes. *(Figure 5)*

AEROBIC WORKOUTS

LET'S TALK MORE ABOUT THE "AEROBIC" and "anaerobic" workouts. During times of rest and low-moderate levels of exercise called aerobic workouts, we don't produce lactic acid.[357] Usually, you can talk during this type of workout. It is highly efficient at producing energy for metabolism.

At this stage, more fat than glucose is burned. Recall that this is the fat burn stage of exercise. As intensity and duration pick up, exercise progresses and there is a gradual shift into the anaerobic phase where mostly glucose is utilized and lactic acid is generated. We become less efficient at utilizing and creating energy; respiratory rate usually becomes very fast at this level and muscle fatigue sets in. For untrained people, the transition from aerobic to anaerobic occurs earlier in the workout, usually when the individual has completed only 40 to 60 percent of the exercise session. As we train our bodies we get better at utilizing our resources. A highly trained individual can be in the aerobic phase for 90 percent of the workout and doesn't build much lactic acid. Then, highly trained athletes feel less fatigue than less well trained people. Higher-intensity workouts can burn more calories, but untrained individuals run the risk of injuries and shorter workouts because they don't use

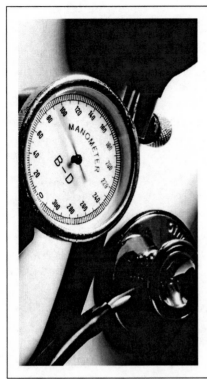

Figure 6:

The Average Shift To Anaerobic Metabolism

Maximum predicted heart rate = 220-age

Most people shift to anaerobic metabolism at 85% of their maximum predicted heart rate

AGE	85% of MPHR
20 *years old*	**170** *heart rate*
30	**162**
40	**153**
50	**145**
60	**136**
70	**128**
80	**119**

oxygen efficiently, which can cause early fatigue.

This is why training is so important, because improved fitness leads to more efficient use of resources and better energy utilization. We can measure endurance and energy utilization through maximal oxygen uptake testing (VO2 max tests). These tests allow us to see a person's maximum ability to utilize oxygen and when she enters the anaerobic phase. These tests require facility testing and are often useful for highly competitive athletes who are trying to maximize efficiency.

For people not interested in the facility testing, a quick way to tell if someone is entering the anaerobic phase is to look at their breathing. When breathing gets more labored (when you cannot talk during exercise), it usually means lactic acid is accumulating; the body is going into the anaerobic phase and is trying to blow off the CO_2 and get more oxygen into the body. The average shift to anaerobic metabolism occurs at about 85% of maximum predicted heart rate (MPHR). Maximum predicted heart rate is determined by the number 220 minus your age. *(Figure 6)* However, many factors impact your transition, specifically your level of training, fitness and nutrient resources available.

"WHAT HEART RATE SHOULD
I AIM FOR, TO BURN THE MOST FAT?"

AGAIN, THIS VARIES FROM PERSON TO PERSON according to their fitness and nutrient status. We know that most fat burn happens below our anaerobic threshold, which is when our bodies utilize fat for energy. Studies show that maximum fat burning occurs between 50 to 80 percent of MPHR.[358] Then a good fat burning goal is to aim for 70 percent of MPHR. Wearing a heart rate monitor is helpful in getting to that goal. One usually can talk through the workout up to that point. Working out at higher levels puts us into an anaerobic zone and causes our breathing to be labored, but we also utilize more glucose than fat with anaerobic exercise. It becomes a great cardiovascular workout but not a fat burn work out. Training can increase fitness levels which increase our ability to break down fat for longer periods of the workout. One study shows that as fitness level improves, fat burning continues at higher heart rates as well.[359]

Varying workout intensity and incorporating both high- and low-intensity workouts in a given week can help you to optimize your fat burning. Someone just starting aerobic exercise should start at 50 to 60 percent of their maximum heart rate as a goal and work on increasing their duration before increasing intensity. Cardiovascular benefits increase with workouts that get us in the anaerobic zone. A gradual increase in intensity will facilitate better tolerance and getting into higher aerobic zones. It is important to discuss the safety of participating in activities that require endurance with your health care provider since the longer and more intense the workouts, the more your heart is taxed.

SWIMMING

AN INCREDIBLE EXERCISE that we have learned to love is swimming. Swimming is the fourth most popular sports activity and is an excellent tool for endurance and resistance. It is often preferred by those who have chronic muscle or joint pain. [360] Studies have shown that in people with rheumatoid arthritis and osteoarthritis, swimming improves the joints without worsening symptoms.[361, 362] This benefit can lead to better endurance in those who have other chronic medical problems as well. Many people have significant concerns with swimming. There are body images issues. We hear often in our clinics about how people would not be "caught dead in a swimsuit." There are also a lot of people who can't swim or aren't confident with their swimming. We remind people that no one really cares what you look like in the pool. Most of us are our own worst critics and at least you are out there doing something! Even if you cannot swim, walking in the pool has benefit.

What about the "I can't swim" issue? Swimming pools always have a shallow section where you can just jump and move. It is amazing how many calories you can lose without realizing it. You will also feel alive. It is an amazing feeling. Dr. A has a patient she has asked to go into the pool for 10 months. Dr. A talked to her about her high blood pressure, significant joint aches and shortness of breath. Ten months later, the patient finally got into a pool. She feels great. Her joints are better. She is walking further and her blood pressure started to finally go down. She gets mad if Dr. A is running late because it cuts into her swimming time! At the end of the day, ongoing physical activity leads to good health.[363] [364]

RESISTANCE EXERCISE.

RESISTANCE EXERCISE IS ALSO CALLED STRENGTH TRAINING. It focuses on building muscle/bone strength, and increases metabolism.[365] The American Heart Association recommends two days of muscle strengthening activity be added to our aerobic workouts. One type of resistance is isotonic exercises. In isotonic exercises, the goal is to work on contracting the muscle by moving the joint and changing the muscle's length. Free weight lifting is an example of isotonic strength training. Lifting weights is a great way to build tone and bulk in muscle. The other type of resistance exercise is isometric

---

Figure 7

Isotonic vs. Isometric

Two types of resistance exercise or strength training—focusing on building muscle/bone strength, and increasing metabolism.

ISOTONIC

Contracting the muscle by moving the joint and changing the muscle length

- Weight lifting
- Pull Ups
- Sit Ups

ISOMETRIC

Contracting the muscle without changing the joint angle or muscle length

- Planks
- Holding a squat
- Fixed yoga poses

exercise. In isometric exercise, the focus of the exercise is contraction of the muscle without changing the joint angle or the muscle length. An example of this is using one's own body weight in a fixed position with weights or with yoga and core exercise. One of our favorite isometric exercises is the plank. *(Figure 7)*

Isometric exercises have therapeutic benefit because they can be done on immobilized limbs, since the joint doesn't need to move. They are of great benefit in older people because the exercises can be done in a seated position with very little space (in a cubicle or wheelchair).[367] Working on contracting muscles such as the pelvic floor, gluteal and abdominal muscles for fixed periods can add up, even when you do them for a few minutes at a time, several times a day during an 8-hour work day.

BENEFITS OF CONDITIONING.

AS THE BODY TRAINS, it becomes more conditioned. Conditioning refers to the concept that the cardiovascular system adapts to increased requirements and demands of exercise and allows the heart to work more efficiently. There is more stroke volume (amount of blood per heart beat) and increased output from the heart. With training, the capacity of the cells increases and cells are able to deliver more oxygen to the rest of the body. As we train, our heart rates go down and resting blood pressure decreases. In addition, the energy producers of our cells, the mitochondria have been found to increase in number with training.[368] With increased mitochondria, we become more energy efficient.

With long-term training we also see the heart hypertrophy or build muscle (not be to be confused with hypertensive heart disease). The heart will also dilate or get bigger in size with endurance exercise. Lung volume also increases. [369]When researchers studied Olympic medalists, they found an increase in survival compared to their age-matched groups from the general population.[370]

Exercise training has the potential to bring about many positive changes to the body. The intensity of the exercise needs to be high enough to activate the body's adaptation response in order to affect the different systems such as metabolism, psychological, endocrine and physiology. If we don't stress the body enough, we will see very little change. Some stress, then, is a good thing – but over time, with overuse, we inflict too much stress on the body and we may develop overuse injury. That can create hormone imbalance, muscle soreness, insomnia and allergenic responses. Recovery from workouts is key. The time between workouts allows for replenishing resources and repair for any tissue injury. Therefore, building endurance must be done over time and slowly.

People often ask which type of cardiovascular exercise is best. The answer is that they are all good. Any exercise that helps us build muscles over time and condition our bodies is good. It is very important to vary workouts and not just focus on aerobic workouts alone.

HORMONES

THERE IS INTERPLAY BETWEEN exercise and hormones. With moderate and intense exercise, cortisol levels increases. Cortisol can inhibit muscle growth and repair and adversely affect our coordination.[371] Cortisol will increase in both fit and unfit individuals with exercise but the levels are higher in an unfit individual. The amount of cortisol rise decreases as fitness increases.[372]

Anabolic hormones (hormones that build muscle) also rise with exercise. Testosterone which is considered an anabolic hormone can help build muscle and support red cells which carry oxygen. Resistance exercise and short term intense interval exercise have shown to elevate testosterone levels. [373] Losing weight with exercise especially abdominal fat, raises testosterone levels as well. Higher testosterone levels also help with recovery. Males, because of their higher testosterone levels, can recover faster than females.[374]

Another anabolic hormone is growth hormone. Growth hormone increases muscle size, increases total body water and not only decreases body fat but also changes the distribution of body fat. Growth hormone levels increase with intensity of the workout and extent of duration of the workout. Moderate prolonged exercise can increase the growth hormone by 10-fold. Data suggest that growth hormone is more associated with peak intensity of exercise than the total work out. Therefore, higher levels of the hormone are associated with harder intensity.[375]

Both testosterone and growth hormone can be regenerative due to their positive effects on muscle and aid in recovery. In cold temperatures, however, both hormones are inhibited and as a result increase recovery time. In addition, as we age, both testosterone and human growth hormone decrease. Exercise then is a nice and natural way to boost both hormones.

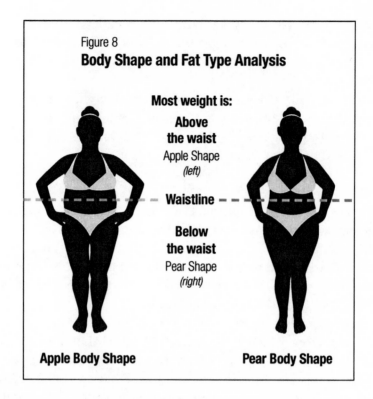

Figure 8
Body Shape and Fat Type Analysis

Most weight is:

Above the waist
Apple Shape
(left)

Waistline

Below the waist
Pear Shape
(right)

Apple Body Shape

Pear Body Shape

HOW DOES EXERCISE AFFECT BODY COMPOSITION?

A COMBINATION OF aerobic exercise and resistance exercise can impact cardiovascular health, and can improve our body composition. Exercise can increase muscle mass and decrease fat percentage, which can be key in managing inflammation and has a direct impact on our immune system.[376] As we discussed, inflammation has a strong connection to many chronic disease states such as diabetes, hypertension, coronary artery disease and cancers. Our bodies have visceral and subcutaneous fat. Visceral fat, or the fat that surrounds our organs, is the most damaging fat to our health because it is inflammatory. Subcutaneous fat, on the other hand, sits right under the skin and is responsible for the "pear shape" fat around the hips and buttocks.

There are two classic body types. One is the "pear shape" fat distribution where fat accumulates around the hips and buttocks. This fat is mostly subcutaneous fat and is of less concern. The "apple shape" fat distribution is more concerning because it is comprised of both visceral and subcutaneous fat *(Figure 8)*.[376] Research shows that this visceral fat can produce inflammatory cytokines (inflammatory chemicals) which alert our bodies that something foreign is present. Other proteins secreted by these fat cells directly result in insulin resistance, elevated blood pressure, altered clotting and alterations in fatty acid metabolism.[377]

This visceral fat also affects our hormonal balance. For example, adrenal hormones such as testosterone can be converted to estrogen in our fat cells. Higher levels of estrogen have been linked to increased risk of postmenopausal breast cancer. There is also an increased conversion from inactive cortisone to active cortisol in our visceral fat. Active cortisol promotes more fat accumulation leading to increasing weight gain which can also propagate further hormone imbalance.[378]. The good news is this visceral fat is more accommodating to lifestyle changes than subcutaneous fat. By lifestyle changes, we mean moderate intense activity along[379] with dietary adjustments more effectively reduces visceral fat than subcutaneous fat. Increasing nutrient-rich foods, and cutting back on calorie-dense foods, can

CONSIDER ❷

The scale can be misleading when you are doing an exercise program. Often with good lifestyle changes, the scale does not change but you will see changes such as loss of inches in the waist and hips

CLINICAL CASE 1: Patient is an avid biker riding over 100 miles per week along with other high intensity workouts per week. She changed her diet to help her pre-diabetes and was still struggling to lose her fat percentage and weight. She had a hamstring injury and could not maintain her high intensity workouts and finally took up yoga and lower intensity workouts. Within a few weeks, she noticed her waist size decrease and her weight reduced by 8 lbs. She felt more energy as well.

HELPFUL TIP: High intensity workouts can become a stressful event for your body. They need to be balanced with lower intensity workouts. Yoga and Pilates are great choices.

CLINICAL CASE 2: Patient had a sedentary lifestyle and started walking around her building for 10,000 steps per day. Along with dietary changes, she lost 15lbs in 6 weeks but then the weight loss stopped. Her body needed more cardiovascular exercise--walking was no longer enough. She then added 3 days of interval training per week and weight loss of 1 lb/week continued.

TAKE HOME: continue to challenge your body with varying workouts.

be a great start. In fact, when vigorous exercise is a regular regimen, it's possible to lose adipose (fatty) tissue without losing weight as you build lean muscle mass.[380] [381]

Several studies have shown that stress is a major contributor to visceral fat and an altered cortisol response.[382] Cortisol is the hormone secreted by our adrenal when we are stressed. We see it in higher levels in those who have health related stress, job stress and school-related stress.[383] In some studies, the stress response has been shown to promote selective visceral fat accumulation and increased insulin resistance.[384] This shows us that stress or cortisol can promote abdominal fat.

Stress to the body can look like sleep deprivation or job, school or family stress, multiple health problems, or very high-intensity exercise. Each person should individualize her approach to reducing fat mass, but when the goal is fat loss, don't ignore the role that stress plays. Stress reduction with a yoga practice, along with breathing techniques, need to be practiced most days. Finding five to 10 minutes a day to meditate, and participating in a yoga class once a week, is a good start to lowering our cortisol levels while following a low-inflammatory diet (see diet section). In addition, looking at insulin resistance, hormone balance and adding nutrient- rich food can all play a role in abdominal weight. Therefore, when you ask, "how do I lose my gut?" there is no easy answer. What we can tell you is to start with a nutrient-rich food plan and combine stress reduction with a balanced workout, including cardiovascular exercise, resistance, balance and stretching. Sometimes working out LESS intensely can lower the stress response and improve abdominal fat. *(Consider 2)*

BROWN ADIPOSE FAT

IT IS INTERESTING TO NOTE that not all body fat is bad for our health. Unlike the white fat, brown adipose tissue (BAT) is a type of fat that boosts our metabolic rate. This rate indicates how much energy we utilize when we're at rest. BAT fat is found in higher amounts in infants and decreases with age. The brown term comes from its high content of mitochondria, the energy producers in our cells. Studies have shown that when brown adipose fat is transplanted into mice, the recipient mice improved their glucose tolerance, increased their insulin sensitivity, lowered their body weight and reduced their fat mass.[385] Researchers publishing in the journal *Nature* in 2012 showed that moderate exercise can transform white adipose tissue into brown adipose tissue and increase metabolic rate and heat production.[386] This suggests that our white adipose tissue can become metabolically trained and more metabolic active.

MOOD

EXERCISE IN THE REALM OF MOOD, sleep restoration, and energy can also make a significant impact. Depression is a common psychiatric disorder. The World Health Organization estimates that more than 350 million people in the world are affected. Finding tools to treat this illness can have a positive global impact. The case in the beginning of the chapter is an example of how exercise can elevate the neurotransmitters (signal messengers) and good energy hormones called endorphins.

Endorphins are opioid like chemicals in our body that can attach to cell receptors and release natural pain killers or analgesics, but can also elevate mood. Studies have shown that endorphins are released when we feel pain and stresses such as exercise.[387] Studies using positron emission tomography (PET scans) have shown specific binding of opioid-like substances in specific areas of the brain following strenuous exercise.[388] Then, exercise can give a high without the harm! Of note, a PET scan is a diagnostic test that utilizes a radioactive tracer that hooks onto a biologically active molecule like a white cell or glucose molecule. It can see the function of tissues instead of just the anatomy.

We release endorphins in direct proportion to our level of exertion, and they act on our brains to create a sense of euphoria. This mechanism is thought to be the reason for a runner's high, which is based on a reward mechanism for prolonged exercise. Endorphins also inhibit the pain response; therefore, the pain of prolonged exercise is often not apparent until after the exercise is finished. Endorphins also raise our pain threshold, which allows us to perform in times of pain.

Neurotransmitters such as serotonin, dopamine and norepinephrine are associated with mood disorders. Many medications used for treating depression target these transmitters. A major review examined 39 different studies to determine the role of exercise in depression. They found that exercise is moderately more effective for reducing symptoms of depression than no therapy at all.[389] Other organizations such as the Association of Medicine and Psychiatry have recommended that primary care doctors strongly advocate exercise to help reduce symptoms in their depressed patients. [390]

One public health study showed group jogging exercise may be effective in improving the outlook of adolescent females with depressive symptoms.[391]The benefits from natural elevation of neurotransmitters, such as mood stabilization and sleep promotion, may eliminate the need for medications in some cases. Exercise provides a potent mood stabilizer without the side effects such as weight gain and sexual dysfunction seen with many medications.

Swiss neuroscientists have also identified a mechanism that protects us from stress-induced depression. A protein call PGC- 1 alpha 1 is known to increase in skeletal muscle with exercise. Researchers conducted a study where they genetically modified mice to have higher levels of PGC- 1 alpha 1 (similar to those with well-trained muscles) and compared them to mice with normal levels of PGC -1 alpha 1. Researchers found when both groups were exposed to stress, the genetically modified mice showed no signs of depression. This change in the genetically modified mice was felt to be due to the impact of exercise on a chemical called kynurenine. Kynurenine is a metabolite of tryptophan, an amino acid involved with mood. This metabolite has been shown to build up during stress. Researchers in this study propose that lowering kynurenine in the blood protects the brain from depression. Skeletal muscles during exercise through PGC -1 alpha 1 pathway reduce kynurenine levels in the blood and create kynurenic acid which is unable to cross from the blood into the brain. They conclude that this mechanism leads to a protective effect against stress-induced depression.[392] Although adding an exercise program should not substitute for counseling or medication in everyone, an integrated program, designed with your provider, can help guide patients on its role in managing mood disorders.

COGNITION.

ONE OF THE MOST EXCITING BENEFITS of aerobic exercise is its role in elevation of Brain Derived Neurotropic Factor (BDNF). It is a protein, located in the brain and made of neurons or nerve cells, and allows for the growth and survival of neurons or nerve cells. The protein helps these cells grow, mature and increase the efficiency of the connection between the neurons. Research shows that BDNF is vital to neuroplasticity, which is the way in which the brain adapts to new challenges in learning and forming memory. Interestingly, BDNF is found in areas of the brain that control eating, drinking and body weight. It's likely that it plays a role in the management of these issues as well. Aerobic exercise has been shown to elevate BDNF levels and improve neuroplasticity.[393] Amazing.

VITAMIN D AND THE SUN

WHEN THE SUN'S UVB RAYS HIT THE SKIN, our skin generates vitamin D. Melanin is a pigment in our skin, protecting it from UVB rays; the darker the skin, the more melanin it contains and the less vitamin D is produced. A light-skinned individual who spends 10 minutes outside makes 25,000 IU of vitamin D, which is very important for mood and many other bodily functions.[415] It's drawn to receptors in the brain, heart, skeletal muscles and immune cells, so it's easy to understand how low levels of vitamin D have been implicated in low mood, poor memory and cardiovascular protection.[416] [417]

IF YOU LIVE AT A LATITUDE NORTH OF ATLANTA, it's difficult to get vitamin D from the sun after August because of the way UVB rays hit the earth. People with fair complexions should check with their providers about their blood levels of vitamin D and the safety of long-term unexposed sun and their personal risk of skin cancer. Gardening is one way of spending time in sunlight and enjoying a healthy activity at the same time.

THERE'S ANOTHER ASPECT OF GARDENING that we don't often think about. Gardening is a physical activity that boosts our heart rate and has a workload of about 4.5-6 METSs. *The American Journal of Public Health* studied health benefits of community gardening and saw that it helped people maintain their healthy body weight. Many gardeners also find great satisfaction in it, aiding their mental health. If you can find an activity you love, such as gardening, you probably will do it more often.

Several studies have looked at improvement in cognition in elderly patients and attribute it to an elevation in BDNF levels. These levels of BDNF were associated with higher levels of physical activity in certain subtypes of patients.[394] Studies have also attributed increases in volumes of different parts of the brain like the hippocampus (a part of our brain which deals with memory), and grey and white matter in the cortex (in charge of higher functions), to elevations in BDNF. In a time when more than 30 percent of Medicare beneficiaries report cognitive impairment or severe dementia, tools like exercise can be very valuable in the prevention of cognitive decline.[395] There are no guarantees, but research shows promise that a regular exercise regimen may help prevent age-related loss of volume in the brain and support cognitive health.[396]

NOVEL WAYS TO EXERCISE

WE OFTEN HEAR, "I don't have time to exercise. Who has an hour to go to the gym?" It is true that an ounce of prevention is worth a pound of treatment – we want to remind readers that even a little goes a long way. In studies, bouts of moderate to intense exercise in 10-minute intervals until you reach 30 minutes a day[397] [398] can still bestow health benefits, especially when someone is first starting to exercise after living a sedentary lifestyle [399] Another novel way to train more efficiently is high-intensity interval training. This is a modality that uses repeated episodes of high intensity from five seconds to eight minutes, followed by varying recovery periods.

You can try this interval training with any endurance activity such as biking, running, cycling and many others. This type of interval training has been shown to improve VO2 max better than continuous moderate intensity training.[400] [401] Recall, improving VO2 max means that our efficiency of using oxygen improves. Higher V02 max in a person suggests improved fitness levels. It also has been shown to reduce fat percentage, [402] and reduce blood pressure and resting heart rate. [403] It causes reductions in biomarkers such as cholesterol, glucose, as well as lowering inflammatory markers of IL-6 and TNF levels.[404] The reason for this benefit is believed to be based on the premise that the exercise intensity is varied but the total energy expenditure of the work out increases.

Tabata is a popular method of high intensity interval training (HIIT), which utilizes 20 seconds of high-intensity exercise alternated with 10 seconds of rest. This is repeated eight times for a total of four minutes. This technique is available also through a phone application called "Tabata" in which you can use to devise your own HIIT workout. This form of workout can last anywhere from 20 to 60 minutes based on fitness level, but it has been shown that energy expenditure from this type of workout is higher than from strict endurance training. It allows our bodies to work out at higher heart rates which is better for our heart and fitness but lowers our injury potential since we are balancing it with lower intensity. Studies show promise for this type of workout regimen; however, further studies are needed to show long term benefits. More importantly, no adverse effects have been reported. This workout also typically lowers high-impact risk to joints and produces fewer injuries since the time spent in high-intensity workouts is less.[405]

When one of our clients, Jane, performs her interval training, a pace of 6 mph is a sprint pace for her. She runs at 6 mph for one minute and then does 4.5 mph for three minutes. She repeats this cycle for a 20-minute workout. According to published studies, she expends more energy with this workout than if she were doing a 4.5-mph jog for 20 minutes, and she would be unlikely to sustain a 6-mph run for 20 minutes because she would push her limits of endurance into high intensity at that pace. If her son, an avid runner, were to do this interval workout, he would run one minute at 9 mph with a jog at 7 mph. You can see how this system depends on your fitness and endurance. The concept is the same but the intensity varies.

STRETCHING AND BALANCE.

STRETCHING AND BALANCE WORK also are integral forms of exercise. Stretching induces flexibility (the ability to move a joint through its complete range of motion). Working on flexibility allows for utilizing the working function of a muscle as long as possible. With muscles, we must "use it or lose it;" we need to reinforce them to maintain their strength.

Balance helps prevent falls and injuries during other activities. It is likely the most undervalued and underutilized component of fitness. As we age, our body changes: we see a decrease in muscle mass and our sensation in our extremities decreases. Another loss is in our vestibular system in our inner ear. The vestibular system coordinates information from our senses and nerves and tells our brain about motion, spatial orientation and aids in our balance. These changes with aging increase our predisposition to falling.

Exercises such as Tai chi and Qigong, types of meditative movement along with yoga, have been shown to improve physical function, flexibility and balance.[406] They often impact positively on quality of life for those with chronic disease, improve pain and movement in people with osteoarthritis, and help to remedy fatigue and depression. Tai chi and Qigong are very similar. They are part of Traditional Chinese Medicine (TCM) and focus on posture and movement, breath, and meditative components. They are considered gentle exercises which employ slow, meditative, flowing dance-like motions.[407] Similarly to yoga, the two forms work on the mind/body connection to help with mood, sleep, flexibility and balance, and help to counter osteoarthritis and osteoporosis.

BENEFIT OF ADDING A FOOD PLAN WITH EXERCISE.

WHEN LOOKING AT THE ROLE OF EXERCISE in weight loss, exercise prescription is often the only lifestyle recommendation patients receive, along with "change your diet." But why should you alter your diet? It is commonly known that exercise can be an integral part of weight management by reducing fat percentage and building muscle mass. Exercise is also touted for its role in supporting bone density, and an asset that helps lower risk of cardiovascular disease and diabetes. While exercise is important for nitric oxide release and weight loss, it doesn't have as much impact without any dietary modification. With exercise alone, you can expect to see about a 2- to 6-percent short-term weight loss (in less than six months). [408] Is that enough? What would happen if we added diet changes. Let's do the math. A pound is equal to 3,500 calories. According to the Calorie Counsel, most Americans consume 4,500 calories on Thanksgiving Day. *The New England Journal of Medicine (NEJM)* states that Americans gain about one pound over the holidays; however, other sources claim the gain is as high as five pounds. Consider, then, that over five years, a person could gain five to 25 pounds just over the holiday season. During the holidays, sugar control also became extremely abnormal.[409] Then, along with weight gain, people were experiencing worsening sugar control. So even if we lose 2- to 6- percent of weight with exercise alone, we will never be effective overall unless we change our diets.

EXERCISE AND BONE LOSS.

ONE MAJOR ILLNESS THAT AFFECTs more people than cardiovascular disease and cancer is osteoporosis or thinning of the bones, which creates a high risk of fragility fracture. Fifty percent of women in menopause will get osteoporosis. Twenty percent of those diagnosed with osteoporosis are men. A hip fracture is more dangerous than it seems; it results in a very high mortality rate due to inactivity, loss of function, infection risk and potential clot formation in the immobile limb. It is critical we have tools to prevent bone loss and do weight-bearing exercises such as weight lifting, walking, running and yoga. High-impact exercises can build bone while low-impact can keep bones strong as well.[410] Strengthening exercises such as weights and yoga can work on muscle strength and balance, which is important for preventing falls.

CANCER PREVENTION.

REGULAR PHYSICAL EXERCISE has been scientifically proven to help prevent cancers. Extensive studies have been conducted regarding breast and colorectal cancers, showing that the more we exercise, the lower our cancer risk. [411] In addition, we know there is a relationship between exercise and a reduction in endometrial, prostate, and lung cancers. Even with a cancer diagnosis, exercise has shown to help increase survivorship by 50 to 60 percent, again with the greatest impact on breast and colorectal cancers.[412] In a study of prostate cancer patients, adding exercise to chemotherapy regimens was found to offset consequences of therapies which inhibit testosterone to decrease tumor size.

These chemotherapy regimens block testosterone and decrease testosterone's ability to grow prostate cancer. Suppressing testosterone, however, can result in lower muscle mass, decreased functional performance and decreased cardiorespiratory fitness. However,researchers showed that in this population, when exercise was added, the cancer did not grow and the side effects were also avoided.[413]

Estrogen can also form into different metabolites. Some of these metabolites are more protective against breast cancers than others.[154] In one study, those who performed 30 minutes of moderate to vigorous aerobic exercise five times per week showed better levels of a more protective estrogen metabolite than the group who led a sedentary lifestyle =GOOD THING.[414]

Recall, higher fat percentage can increase estrogen. So losing fat percentage with exercise can reduce estrogen levels that could be cancer promoting=GOOD THING.

Is running the only exercise? Absolutely *not*. We can name plenty of exercises that don't involve that kind of impact. Walking, swimming and yoga are all great exercises. Gardening is another fine activity with both cardiovascular and resistance benefits, and it also has been found to improve mood, allows us to get creative, and gives us a sense of accomplishment – and working outside in the sunlight (and soaking up vitamin D) and fresh air help us as well.

PLAY.

WHILE EXERCISE IS SO IMPORTANT to maintaining a positive mood, other important activities require less endurance than an exercise regimen, but they still enhance your health. Consider exercise that really is play, and how it affects your mood. We forget how a simple walk in the rain, jumping in puddles, and impromptu dancing with family elevates our mood by movement, and they also awaken our childhood responses of being playful and uninhibited. Taking the competition out of sports and having a friendly game of basketball, softball or Frisbee in the outdoors is also exercise.

Adults tend to forget the role of free play because we are so focused on tasks and being responsible. Playing in the yard with pets or kids, making a snowman, pillow fighting, running in the yard and blowing bubbles are all examples of activities that raise your heart rate. Even a game of very enthusiastic charades can be both physical activity but also great for your mental health. If you can find a physical activity that you also enjoy, you can easily make it a regular part of your life.

Along with joyful play, the role of laughter also has been studied. We know how good laughter can make us feel. Studies have shown that laughter can give us joy by raising our pain threshold, elevating our endorphins and improving our mood, but it also exercises our diaphragm, which is a muscle.[418] Surprisingly, working your diaphragm by simply laughing can be a form of exercise!

Dr. Madan Kataria, a physician from Mumbai, India, devised the concept of "laughter yoga" in 1995. Students begin their "laughter practice" as a structured class that involves movement, deep breathing and stretches, during which the instructor is the only one talking. The instructor guides the students in a 20- to 45-minute class where they learn various laughing techniques. Today, teachers in 60 countries are certified to lead these classes believed to reduce stress and support participants' immune systems while they work on physical activity. Another study which looked at nursing students showed that laughter yoga for two 1-hour sessions per week produced improvement in general health and diminished sleep disorders, lowered anxiety and depression and promoted social function.[419] Voluntary prolonged laughter is thought to have similar benefits of spontaneous laughter. Dr Kataria's website offers locations of laughing clubs in different areas around the world. Imagine how good your mood would be if you started your day after 45 minutes of laughter!

HOW DO I START EXERCISING?

YOU MAY SAY "THAT'S GREAT—there are a lot of benefits to exercise—but how do I start an exercise regimen when I feel so tired all the time?" This is a common question we hear frequently. It can be overwhelming to think of moving 150 minutes a week, as many experts recommend. The goal is to start with 10 minutes. Take a new, longer route from the parking lot to work. Stand and do slow movements during TV commercials, and do Kegel exercises (pelvic floor crunches) while sitting in your chair at work. Play catch with kids or grandkids, or start dancing to music. You can start doing diaphragmatic breathing several times per day.

You will find ways to move. The best part of exercise is, it usually becomes a segue to other healthier habits such as eating more nutrient-rich foods, sleeping more restfully, drinking more water and more.

It is sometimes easier to initiate a new habit when we feel accountable. Try wearing an activity tracker. A variety of products on the market count your steps, evaluate the quality of your sleep, and count calories burned, floors climbed and record the intensity of your activity. You can choose a device that matches your needs.

You can always start with a simple, inexpensive pedometer and monitor your steps. The goal for most people is 10,000 steps per day. You will be shocked at how few steps you take in a day, especially if you have a desk job. People who tell us they walk all the time usually clock between 2,000 to 3,000 steps per day. You also will be surprised when you see how easy it is to increase your steps by going for a walk at lunchtime, parking farther away or taking the stairs instead of riding the elevator.

We have found our patients really respond to knowing their step counts every day because it gives them goals. Get creative. Make exercise social—something fun, an activity you look forward to. Small steps along a new path will take you to a new, fun destination. At the same time, you must learn to walk before you run. Start slowly and build each week. For those who do not walk much, start by walking to the corner of your block several times a day. Then add walking around the block and increase it towards a goal of 30-minute intervals for five minutes per week. You can do this. ▪

10 Recommended Exercises for Alignment/Posture

Exercise usually becomes a segue to other healthier habits

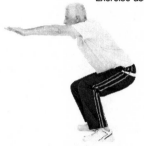

❶ SQUATS: Body weight exercise that primarily targets your thighs (quadriceps, hamstrings), buttocks (gluteal muscles), and calves

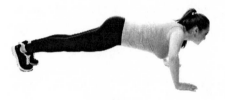

❷ PUSH-UPS: Body Weight exercise that targets your upper body & core (abdominal/back) muscles.

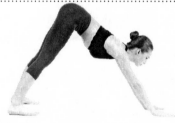

❸ DOWNWARD DOG: stretching and strengthening yoga pose— energizes the body—calms the brain and helps relieve stress.

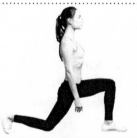

❹ FRONT LUNGE: Focuses on strengthening of the lower body, balance, coordination, and flexibility.

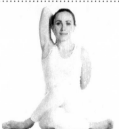

❺ SEATED CHEST STRETCH: Chest Stretch: Improves posture, reduces tight muscles in the chest, and helps to strengthen upper body muscles to reduce kyphosis.

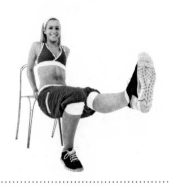

6 **SEATED HIP MARCH:** Strengthens hips and thigh muscles by sitting on the edge of chair and alternate lifting one leg (bent knee) off the floor as high as possible.

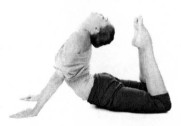

7 **PRONE COBRA:** Lie on your stomach and engage your core as you lift arms out to side and legs up simultaneously

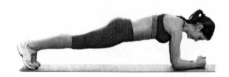

8 **BODY PLANK:** A floor exercise that works your whole body as you fight against gravity, primarily focusing on your core muscles.

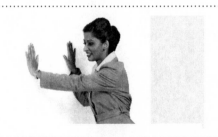

9 **DOOR FRAME STRETCH:** Door Frame Stretch: "Similar to seated chest press", this one you're standing. Stretches out Chest, Shoulders, & Back.

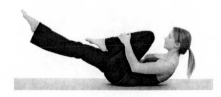

10 **STRAIGHT LEG RAISE:** Lie on your back, lift 1 or 2 legs together will determine the flexibility of hamstrings which can affect posture & alignment and if low back pain is present.

YOUR PRESCRIPTION:

Developing Your Own Exercising Program

1 **Start low and go slow**

2 **Change it up**, continue to challenge yourself, change your workout and intensity as you get stronger

3 **A complete workout is more than just getting your heart rate up.** Add resistance and strengthen your core. Sometimes, balance is as important as aerobics for other health benefits. Recovery is very important too.

4 **Learn to laugh and play!**

CHAPTER 15:

Recharge

Eat well, play more, sleep deeply. Heal.

A HEALTHY BODY IS A BODY IN BALANCE. The balance between eustress and distress; the balance between the sympathetic "fight or flight" and parasympathetic "rest and recharge" systems; the balance between resource depletion and replenishment. We must maintain that balance to be healthy--to achieve homeostasis.

While stress is a normal part of life, most of us have created lives for ourselves in which we are constantly on the go. We are overstimulated by electronics and work. We multitask. We handle large amounts of emotional stress. We eat poorly. We don't sleep enough. We deprive our bodies of that balance and this leads to inflammation and ultimately illness.

Learning how to maintain balance is a true art. Taking time to recharge the body with rest, yoga, meditation and exercise is essential. Eating nourishing foods, slowing down our pace and learning the beauty of taking our time are vital steps to counterbalancing all these depletive sources of stress in our lives. We live in a world where stress is worn as a badge of honor. We are proud of how well we perform on little sleep and how little we need to manage. We are proud of our "go, go, go" and "play hard" mentalities. Ultimately, however, the balance is shifted and we get sick. It is inevitable. It happened to Dr. A and so many others and it will happen to you—unless you change. Change is hard. To so many people, taking the time to rest and recharge is looked at as a sign of weakness.

We argue that that mentality has to change. We choose to take back our lives and we wear our rest and recharge time as our badges of honor-- because without the balance, the body cannot heal.

The process will be slow but each day, take one step. Try to find twenty minutes to deep breathe. Try to put your electronics away fifteen minutes before bed. Try to go for a walk. Try to eliminate processed foods and meats to start. Even with small steps, you will start to feel different—better. Small steps will lead to big steps.

With this book, we give you the tools you need to live your life well, with energy and without illness. This is what we want for you. With the best in mind for you, be well. Nourish your body, your microbiome, and your soul. Rest. Take time to play and sleep. Eat abundantly and well.

Best, Monica and Jyothi

ENDNOTES

CHAPTER 4:

1. Schneiderman N, Ironson G, Siegal SD. Stress and Health: Psychological, behavioral, and biological determinants. Annu Rev Clin Psychol; 2005; 1: 607-628.

2. Schneiderman N, Ironson G, Siegal SD. Stress and Health: Psychological, behavioral, and biological determinants. Annu Rev Clin Psychol .2005; 1: 607-628.

3. Donoho CJ, Weigensberg MJ, Emken BA. Stress and abdominal fat: preliminary evidence of moderation by the cortisol awakening response in Hispanic peripubertal girls. Obesity; May 2011; 19(5): 946-952

4. Donoho CJ, Weigensberg MJ, Emken BA. Stress and abdominal fat: preliminary evidence of moderation by the cortisol awakening response in Hispanic peripubertal girls. Obesity; May 2011; 19 (5):946-952.

5. Schneiderman N, Ironson G, Siegal SD. Stress and Health: psychological, behavioral and biological determinants. Annu Rev Clin Psychol; 2005; 607-628.

6. Schbacher K, O'Donovan A, Wolkowitz O, Dhabhar F, Su Y, Epel E. Good stress, bad stress and oxidative stress: insights from anticipatory cortisol reactivity. Psychoneuroendocrinology; Sept 2013; 38(9): 1698-708.

7. Schbacher K, O'Donovan A, Wolkowitz O, Dhabhar F, Su Y, Epel E. Good stress, bad stress and oxidative stress: insights from anticipatory cortisol reactivity. Psychoneuroendocrinology; Sept 2013; 38(9): 1698-708.

8. Miller GE, Cohen S, Ritchey AK. Chronic psychological stress and the regulation of pro-inflammatory cytokines: a glucocorticoid–resistance model. Health Psychol; Nov. 2002; 21 (6):531-41.

9. Harbuz MS, Chover-Gonzalez AJ, Jessop DS. Hypothalamo-pituitary–adrenal axis and chronic immune activation. Ann. NY Acad Sci 2003; 992: 99-106.

10. Epel E, Blackburn EH, Lin J, Dhabhar FS, Adler NE, Morrow JD, Cawthon RM. Accelerated telomere shortening in response to life stress. PNAS; December 2004; 101 (49): 17312-315.

CHAPTER 5:

11. Top 10 causes of death fact sheet. World Health Organization 5/2014; http://www.who.int/mediacentre/factsheets/fs310/en/

12. Ogden CL, Carroll MD, Kit BK, Flegal KM. Prevalence of childhood and adult obesity in the United States 2011-2012. JAMA; 2014;311(8):806-814.

13. Flegal KM, Carroll MD, Kit BK, Ogden CL. Prevalence of obesity and trends in the distribution of body mass index among US adults, 1999–2010. JAMA; 2012; 307(5):491–97

14. National Diabetes Statistics Report, 2014. http://www.cdc.gov/diabetes

15. Clinical Guidelines on the Identification, Evaluation, and Treatment of Overweight and Obesity in Adults. The Evidence Report. NIH publications. No. 98-4083. September 1998

16. Vogel R, Corretti M, Plotnick GD. Effect of a single high-fat meal on endothelial function in healthy subjects. American Journal of Cardiology; February 1997; 79 (3): 350–354.

17. Enos WF, Holmes RH, Beyer J. Coronary disease among United States soldiers killed in action in Korea: preliminary report. JAMA; 1953; 152: 1090-1093

18. McNamara JJ, Molot MA, Stremple JF, Cutting RT. Coronary artery disease in combat casualties in Vietnam. JAMA; 1971; 216: 1185-1187.

19. Calle E, Rodriguez C, Walker-Thurmond K, Thun MJ. Overweight, obesity, and mortality from cancer in a prospectively studied cohort of U.S. adults. N Engl J Med; 2003; 348:1625-1638.

20. Gallup-Healthways Well-Being Index, 2009

21. Katherine M. Flegal, Brian K. Kit, Heather Orpana, Barry I. Graubard. Association of all-cause mortality with overweight and obesity using standard body mass index: A systematic review and meta-analysis. JAMA; Jan 2013

22. Calle E, Rodriguez C, Walker-Thurmond K, Thun MJ. Overweight, obesity, and mortality from cancer in a prospectively studied cohort of U.S. adults. N Engl J Med; 2003; 348:1625-1638.

23. Prospective Studies Collaboration. Body-mass index and cause-specific mortality in 900,000 adults: collaborative analyses of 57 prospective studies. 2009; Mar 28; 373(9669):1083-96.

24. Goldstein DJ, Beneficial health effects of modest weight loss, Int J Obes Relat Metab Disord. June 1992: 397-415.

25. CDC. Vital signs: prevalence, treatment, and control of high levels of low-density lipoprotein cholesterol. United States, 1999–2002 and 2005–2008. MMWR; 2011; 60(4):109–14.

26. Nwankwo T, Yoon SS, Burt V, Gu Q. Hypertension among adults in the US: national health and nutrition examination survey, 2011-2012 NCHS Data Brief, No. 133. Hyattsville, MD: National Center for Health Statistics, Centers for Disease Control and Prevention, US Dept of Health and Human Services, 2013.

27. Hubert HB, Feinleib M, McNamara PM, Castelli WP. Obesity as an independent risk factor for cardiovascular disease: a 26-year follow-up of participants in the Framingham Heart Study. Circulation; 1983; 67: 968-97.

28. Danner FW. A national longitudinal study of the association between hours of TV viewing and the trajectory of BMI growth among US children. J Pediatr Psychol; 2008; 33: 1100-7

CHAPTER 6:

29. Stilling RM, Dinan TG, Cryan JF. Microbial genes, brain and behavior-epigenetic regulation of the gut-brain axis. Genes, Brain and Behavior; 2014; 13:69-86.

30. Robinson CJ, Bohannan BJM, Young VB. From structure to function: the ecology of host-associated microbial communities. Microbiology and Molecular Biology Reviews; September 2010; 74(3): 453-6.

31. Cho I, Blaser MJ. The Human Microbiome: at the interface of health and disease. Nat Rev Genet; 2012; 13(4): 260–270.

32. Stilling RM, Dinan TG, Cryan JF. Microbial genes, brain and behavior-epigenetic regulation of the gut-brain axis. Genes, Brain and Behavior; 2014; 13:69-86.

33. Stilling RM, Dinan TG, Cryan JF. Microbial genes, brain and behavior-epigenetic regulation of the gut-brain axis. Genes, Brain and Behavior; 2014; 13:69-86.

34. Stilling RM, Dinan TG, Cryan JF. Microbial genes, brain and behavior-epigenetic regulation of the gut-brain axis. Genes, Brain and Behavior; 2014; 13:69-86.

35. Critchfield JW, Van Hemert S, Ash M, Mulder L, Ashwood P. The Potential Role of Probiotics in the Management of Childhood Autism Spectrum Disorders. Gastroenterology Research and Practice; 2011; 201.

36. Falk PG, Hooper LV, Midtvedt T, Gordon JI. Creating and maintaining the gastrointestinal ecosystem: what we know and need to know from gnotobiology. Microbiol Mol Biol Rev; 1988; 62:1157–70.

37. Hooper LV, Gordon JI. Commensal host-bacterial relationships in the gut. Science; 292:1115–1118.

38. Blaser MJ. Who are we? Indigenous microbes and the ecology of human diseases. EMBO; 2006; Rep 7:956–960.

39. Strachan DP. Hay fever, hygiene, and household size. BMJ; 1989; 299:1259– 1260.

40. Macfarlane S, Macfarlane GT. Regulation of short-chain fatty acid production. Proc Nutr Soc; 2003; 62: 67-72.

41. De Filippo C, Cavalieri D, Di Paola M, Ramazzotti M, Poullet JB, Massart S, Collini S, Pieraccini G, Lionetti P. Impact of diet in shaping gut microbiota revealed by a comparative study in children from Europe and rural Africa. PNAS; 2010; 107: 14691–14696.

42. De Filippo C, Cavalieri D, Di Paola M, Ramazzotti M, Poullet JB, Massart S, Collini S, Pieraccini G, Lionetti P. Impact of diet in shaping gut microbiota revealed by a comparative study in children from Europe and rural Africa. PNAS; 2010;107: 14691–14696.

43. Zhang H, DiBaise JK, Zuccolo A, Kudrna D, Braidotti M, Yu Y, Parameswaran P, Crowell MD, Wing R, Rittmann BE, Krajmalnik-Brown R. Human gut microbiota in obesity and after gastric bypass. Proceedings of the National Academy of Sciences of the United States of America; 2009; 106(7):2365–70.

44. Kondo S, Xiao JZ, Satoh T, Odamaki T, Takahashi S, Sugahara H, Yaeshima T, Iwatsuki K, Kamei A, Abe K. Antiobesity effects of Bifidobacterium breve strain B-3 supplementation in a mouse model with high-fat diet-induced obesity. Bioscience, Biotechnology, and Biochemistry; 2010; 74(8):1656–1661.

45. Maslowski KM, Vieira AT, Ng A, Kranich J, Sierro F, Yu D, Schilter HC, Rolph MS, Mackay F, Artis D, Xavier RJ, Teizeira MM, Mackay CR. Regulation of inflammatory responses by gut microbiota and chemoattractant receptor GPR43. Nature; 2009; 461:1282–1286.

46. Vinolo MAR, Rodriques HG et al., Regulation of inflammation by short chain fatty acids. Nutrients; Oct 2011; 3(10): 858-876.

47. Cummings JH. Short-chain fatty acid enemas in the treatment of distal ulcerative colitis. Open Biochem J; 2010; 4: 53–58.

48. Vinolo MA, Rodrigues HG, Hatanaka E, Sato FT, Sampaio SC, Curi R. Suppressive effect of short-chain fatty acids on production of proinflammatory mediators by neutrophils. J Nutr Biochem; 2011;22:849–855.

49. Olefsky JM, Glass CK. Macrophages, inflammation, and insulin resistance. Annu Rev.Physiol; 2010; 72:219–246.

50. Kinne RW, Brauer R, Stuhlmuller B, Palombo-Kinne E, Burmester GR. Macrophages in rheumatoid arthritis. Arthritis Res; 2000; 2:189–202

51. Waldecker M, Kautenburger T, Daumann H, Busch C, Schrenk D. Inhibition of histone-deacetylase activity by short-chain fatty acids and some polyphenol metabolites formed in the colon. J Nutr Biochem 2008;19: 587–93.

52. Wold KJ, Lorenz RG. Gut Microbiota and Obesity. Curr Obes Rep; March 2012; 1(1): 18.

53. Wold KJ, Lorenz RG. Gut Microbiota and Obesity. Curr Obes Rep; March 2012; 1(1): 18.

54. Berk M, Williams LJ, Jacka FN, O'Neil AO, Pasco JA, Moylan S, Allen NB, Stuart AL, Hayley AC, Byrne ML, Maes M. So depression is an inflammatory disease, but where does the inflammation come from? BMC Medicine; 11:200, 1-16.

55. Pussinen PJ, Havulinna AS, Lehto M, Sundvall J, Salomaa V. Endotoxemia is associated with an increased risk of incident diabetes. Diabetes Care; 2011; 34(2):392–397.

56. Naito E, Yoshida Y, Makino K, Kounoshi Y, Kunihiro S, Takahashi R, Matzuzaki T, Miyazaki K, Ishikawa F. Beneficial effect of oral administration of lactobacillus casei strain shirota on insulin resistance in diet-induced obesity mice. Journal of Applied Microbiology; 2011; 110(3):650–657.

57. Zhang R et al., J Neuroimmunol; 2009; (206): 121-4.

58. Emanuele E et al., Neuroscience Letters; 2010; 471: 162-5.

59. Meek TH, Morton GJ. Leptin, diabetes, and the brain. Indian J Endocrinol; 2012 Dec; 16 (Suppl 3): S534–S542.

60. Martin G. Myers, Jr., Steven B. Heymsfield, Carol Haft, Barbara B. Kahn, Maren Laughlin, Rudolph L. Leibel, Matthias H. Tschöp, Jack A. Yanovski, and the attendees of the NIH conference. Toward a Clinical Definition of Leptin Resistance: Defining clinical leptin resistance—challenges and opportunities. Cell Metabolism; 2012; 15(2): 150–156.

61. Zhang Y, Proenca R, Maffei M, Barone M, Leopold L, Friedman JM. Positional cloning of the mouse obese gene and its human homologue. Nature; 1994; 372:425–32.

62. Halaas JL, Gajiwala KS, Maffei M, Cohen SL, Chait BT, Rabinowitz D, Lallone RL, Burley SK, Friedman JM. Weight-reducing effects of the plasma protein encoded by the obese gene. Science; 1995; 269:543–6.

63. Considine RV, Sinha MK, Heiman ML, Kriauciunas A, Stephens TW, Nyce MR, Ohannesian JP, Marco CC, McKee LJ, Bauer TL, Caro JF. Serum immunoreactive-leptin concentrations in normal-weight and obese humans. N Engl J Med; 1996; 334:292–295

64. Shapiro A, Mu W, Roncal C, Cheng KY, Johnson RJ, Scarpace PJ. Fructose-induced leptin resistance exacerbates weight gain in response to subsequent high-fat feeding. Am J Physiol Regul Integr Comp Physiol; Nov 2008; 295(5): R1370–R1375.

65. Tang WH, Wang Zeneng et al., Intestinal Microbial Metabolism of Phosphatidylcholine and Cardiovascular Risk. N Engl J Med; 2013; 368: 1575-84.

66. Stilling RM, Dinan TG, Cryan JF. Microbial genes, brain and behavior-epigenetic regulation of the gut-brain axis. Genes, Brain and Behavior; 2014; 13:69-86.

67. Vaarala O. Leaking gut in type 1 diabetes. Curr Opin Gastroenterol; 2008; 24(6): 701-6.

68. Berk M, Williams LJ, Jacka FN, O'Neil AO, Pasco JA, Moylan S, Allen NB, Stuart AL, Hayley AC, Byrne ML, Maes M. So depression is an inflammatory disease, but where does the inflammation come from? BMC Medicine; 11:200, 1-16.

69. Berk M, Williams LJ, Jacka FN, O'Neil AO, Pasco JA, Moylan S, Allen NB, Stuart AL, Hayley AC, Byrne ML, Maes M. So depression is an inflammatory disease, but where does the inflammation come from? BMC Medicine; 11:200, 1-16.

70. Cani PD, Bibiloni R, Knauf C, Waget A, Neyrinck AM, Delzenne NM, Burcelin R. Changes in gut microbiota control metabolic endotoxemia-induced inflammation in high-fat diet-induced obesity and diabetes in mice. Diabetes; 2008; 57(6):1470–1481.

71. Vaziri ND. CKD impairs barrier function and alters microbial flora of the intestine: a major link to inflammation and uremic toxicity. Nov 2012;21(6):587-92.

72. O'Keefe SJ, Lahti L, Ou J, Carbonero F, Mohammed K, Posma JM, Kinross J, Wahl E, Ruder E, Vipperla K, Naidoo V, Mtshali L, Tims S, Puylaert PG, DeLany J, Krasinskas A, Benefiel AC, Kaseb HO, Newton K, Nicholson JK, de Vos WM, Gaskins HR, Zoetendal EG. Fat, fibre and cancer risk in African Americans and rural Africans. Nature Communications; Jan 2015; Article 6342.

73. Ichinohe T, Pang IK, Kumamoto Y, Peaper DR, Ho JH, Murray TS, Iwasaki A. Microbiota regulates immune defense against respiratory tract influenza A virus infection. Proc Natl Acad Sci USA; 2011; 108:5354–59.

74. Guandalini S, Pensabene L, Zikri MA, Dias JA, Casali LG , Hoekstra H , Kolacek S , Massar K , Micetic-Turk D , Papadopoulou A , de Sousa JS , Sandhu B , Szajewska H , Weizman Z. Lactobacillus GG administered in oral rehydration solution to children with acute diarrhea: a multicenter European trial. J Pediatr Gastroenterol Nutr; 30:54–60.

75. Hui AWH, Lau HW, Chan TH, Tsui SK. The human microbiota: a new direction in the investigation of thoracic diseases. J Thorac Dis; August 2013; 5: S127-S131.

76. vanNood E, Vrieze A, Nieuwdorp M, Fuentes S, Zoetendal EG, de Vos WM, Visser CE, Kuijper EJ, Bartelsman JF, Tijssen JG, Speelman P, Dijkgraaf MG, Keller JJ, Duodenal infusion of donor feces for recurrent Clostridium difficile. NEJM; Jan 2013; 368:407-415.

77. Salminen S, Gibson C, Bouley MC, Isolauri E, Boutron-Rualt MC, Cummings J, Franck A, Rowland I, Roberfroid M. Gastrointestinal physiology and function: the role of prebiotics and probiotics. Br J Nutr. 1998; 80(Suppl 1):S147-71.

78. Savaiano DA, Abou EA, Smith DE, Levitt MD. Lactose malabsorption from yogurt, sweet acidophilus milk, and cultured milk in lactose deficient individuals. Am J Clin Nutr; 1984; 40:1219–23.

79. Goldin BR, Gorbach SR. Clinical indications for probiotics: an overview. Clinical Infectious Diseases; 2008; 46:S96–100

80. Guandalini S, Pensabene L, Zikri MA, et al., Lactobacillus GG administered in oral rehydration solution to children with acute diarrhea: a multicenter European trial. J Pediatr Gastroenterol Nutr; 2000; 30:54–60.

81. Hilton E, Kolakowski P, Singer C, Smith M. Efficacy of lactobacillus GG as a diarrheal preventive in travelers. J Travel Med; 1997; 4:41–3.

82. Kalliomaki M, Salminen S, Arvilommi H, Kero P, Koskinen P, Isolauri E. Probiotics in primary prevention of atopic disease: a randomized placebo-controlled trial. Lancet; 2001; 357:1076–9.

83. Goldin BR, Gorbach SR. Clinical indications for probiotics: an overview. Clinical Infectious Diseases; 2008; 46:S96–100

84. Hatakka K, Martio J, Korpela M, Herranen M, Poussa T, Laasanen T, Saxelin M, Vapaatalo H, Moilanen E, Korpela R: Effects of probiotic therapy on the activity and activation of mild rheumatoid arthritis-a pilot study. Scand J Rheumatol; 2003, 32: 211–215.

85. Mandel DR, Eickas K et al., *Bacillus coagulans:* a viable adjunct therapy for relieving symptoms of rheumatoid arthritis according to a randomized, controlled trial. BMC Complement Altern Med; 2010; 10: 1.86,

CHAPTER 7:

86. Wilson Tang WH, Wang Z, Levison BS, Koeth RA, Britt EB, Fu X, Wu Y, Hazen SL. Intestinal Microbial Metabolism of Phosphatidylcholine and Cardiovascular Risk. N Engl J Med 2013; 368: 1575-1584.

87. Pan A, Sun Q, Bernstein AM, Schulze MB, Manson JE, Stampfer MJ, Willett WC, Hu FB. Red meat consumption and mortality results from 2 prospective cohort studies. Arch Intern Med, 2012;172(7):555-563

88. Kleinbongard P, Dejam A, Lauer T, Jax T, Kerber S, Gharini P, Balzer J, Zotz RB, Scharf RE, Willers R, Schechter AN, Feelisch M, Kelm M. Plasma nitrite concentrations reflect the degree of endothelial dysfunction in humans. Free Radic Biol Med. 2006; 40(2): 295-302.

89. Pereira EC, Ferderbar S, Bertolami MC, Faludi AA, Monte O, Javier HT, Pereira TV, Abdalla DS. Biomarkers of oxidative stress and endothelial dysfunction in glucose intolerance and diabetes mellitus. Clin Biochem. 2008; 41(18): 1454-1460

90. Esselstyn CB, Gendy G, Doyle J, Golubic M, Roizen MF. A way to reverse CAD? Journal of Family Practice. July 2014; 63(7): p356-36b

91. Pan A, Sun Q, Bernstein AM, Schulze MB, Manson JE, Stampfer MJ, Willett WC, Hu FB. Red Meat consumption and mortality results from 2 prospective cohort studies. Arch Intern Med, 2012; 172(7): 555-563

92. Skog K, Steineck G, Augustsson K, Jägerstad M. Effect of cooking temperature on the formation of heterocyclic amines in fried meat products and pan residues. Carcinogenesis, 1995; 16(4): 861-867

93. Cross AJ, Pollock JR, Bingham SA. Haem, not protein or inorganic iron, is responsible for endogenous intestinal N-nitrosation arising from red meat. Cancer Res. 2003; 63(10): 2358-2360

94. Pan A, Sun Q, Bernstein AM, Schulze MB, Manson JE, Stampfer MJ, Willett WC, Hu FB. Red meat consumption and mortality results from 2 prospective cohort studies. Arch Intern Med; 2012; 172(7): 555-563

95. Cerqueira MT, Fry MM, Connor WE. The food and nutrient intakes of the Tarahumara Indians of Mexico. Am J Clin Nutr, 1979; 32: 905-915.

96. Cerqueira MT, Fry MM, Connor WE. The food and nutrient intakes of the Tarahumara Indians of Mexico. Am J Clin Nutr, 1979; 32: 905-915.

97. Kromhout D, Bosschieter EB, Coulander CdL. The inverse relation between fish consumption and 20-year mortality from coronary heart disease. N Engl J Med, 1985; 312: 1205-1209.

98. Marckmann P, Gronbaek M. Fish consumption and coronary heart disease mortality: a systematic review of prospective cohort studies. Eur J Clin Nutr. 1999; 53: 585-90.

99. Campbell T. The China Study. BenBella Books, Inc; 2006.

100. Deopurkar R, Ghanim H, Friedman J, Abuaysheh S, Sia CL, Mohanty P, Viswanathan P, Chaudhuri A, Dandona P. Differential effects of cream, glucose, and orange juice on inflammation, endotoxin, and the expression of Toll-like receptor-4 and suppressor of cytokine signaling-3. Diabetes Care, May 2010; 33(5): 991-7.

101. Cui X, Zuo P, Zhang Q, Li X, Hu Y, Long J, Cui X, Packer L, Liu J. Chronic systemic D-galactose exposure induces memory loss, neurodegeneration, and oxidative damage in mice: protective effects of R-alpha-lipoic acid. J Neurosci Res; 2006; 83: 1584-90.

102. Cui X, Zuo P, Zhang Q, Li X, Hu Y, Long J, Cui X, Packer L, Liu J. Chronic systemic D-galactose exposure induces memory loss, neurodegeneration, and oxidative damage in mice: protective effects of R-alpha-lipoic acid. J Neurosci Res; 2006; 83: 1584-90.

103. Michaëlsson K, Wolk A, Langenskiöld S, Basu S, Lemming EW, Melhus H, Byberg L. Milk intake and risk of mortality and fractures in women and men: cohort studies. BMJ; 2014; 349: g6015.

104. Sonestedt E, Wirfalt E, Wallstrom P, Gullberg B, Orho-Melander M, Hedblad B. Dairy products and its association with incidence of cardiovascular disease: the Malmo diet and cancer cohort. Eur J Epidemiol; 2011; 26: 609-18.

105. Huth PJ, Park KM. Influence of dairy product and milk fat consumption on cardiovascular disease risk: a review of the evidence. Adv Nutr; 2012; 3: 266-85.

106. Michaëlsson K, Wolk A, Langenskiöld S, Basu S, Lemming EW, Melhus H, Byberg L. Milk intake and risk of mortality and fractures in women and men: cohort studies. BMJ; 2014; 349: g6015.

107. Feskanich D, Willett WC, Stamper MJ, Colditz GA. Milk, dietary calcium, and bone fractures in women: a 12-year prospective study. Am J Pub Health; June 1997, 87 (6): 992-7.

108. Feskanich D, Willett WC, Stamper MJ, Colditz GA. Milk, dietary calcium, and bone fractures in women: a 12-year prospective study. Am J Pub Health; June 1997, 87 (6): 992-7.

109. Bischoff-Ferrari HA, Baron, JA, Burckhardt P, Ruifeng L, Spiegelman D, Specker B, Orav JR, Wong JB, Staehelin HB, Reilly EO, Kiel DP, Willett WC. Calcium intake and hip fracture risk in men and women: a meta-analysis of prospective cohort studies and randomized control trials. Am J Clin Nutr, 2007; 86(6): 1780-90.

110. Weaver, C, Plawecki, K. Dietary calcium adequacy of a vegetarian diet. American Journal of Clinical Nutrition; 1994; 1238S-41S.

111. Feskanich D, Willett WC, Stamper MJ, Colditz GA. Protein consumption and bone fractures in women. Am J Epidemiol. 1996; 143: 472–79.

112. Dietary guidelines at http://www.health.gov/dietaryguidelines/dga2005/document/html/appendixB.htm

113. Heaner RP, Weaver CM. Calcium absorption from kale. AJCN; 1990; 51: 656-7.

114. Calcium and milk: what's best for your bones and health? The Nutrition Source, Harvard School of Public Health.

115. Feskanich D, Weber P, Willett WC, Rockett H, Booth SL, Colditz GA. Vitamin K intake and hip fractures in women: a prospective study. Am J Clin Nutr. 1999; 69: 74-79.

116. Booth SL, Tucket KL et al., Dietary vitamin K intakes are associated with hip fracture but not with bone mineral density in elderly men and women. Am J Cl Nutr. 2000; 71: 1201-08.

117. Lampe JW. Dairy products and cancer. J Am Coll Nutr 2011; 30(5 Suppl 1): 464S-70S.

118. Genkinger JM, Hunter DJ, Spiegelman D, Anderson KE, Arslan A, Beeson WL, Buring JE, Fraser GE, Freudenheim JL, Goldbohm RA, Hankinson SE, Jacobs DR Jr. Dairy products and ovarian cancer: a pooled analysis of 12 cohort studies. Cancer Epidemio Biomarkers Prev. 2006; 15: 364-72.

119. Giovannuvvi E, Rimm EB. Calcium and fructose intake in relation to risk of prostate cancer. Cancer Res; 1998; 58: 442-447.

120. Giovannucci E, Liu Y, Platz EA, Stampfer MJ, Willett WC. Risk factors for prostate cancer incidence and progression in the Health Professionals Follow-up Study. International Journal of Cancer; 2007; 121: 1571-78.

121. Danby FW. Nutrition and Acne. Clinics in Dermatology; November–December 2010; 28 (6): 598–604.

122. Campbell, T. The China Study. BenBella Books, Inc. 2006, p. 60-61.

123. Michaëlsson K, Wolk A, Langenskiöld S, Basu S, Lemming EW, Melhus H, Byberg L ,Milk intake and risk of mortality and fractures in women and men: cohort studies. BMJ; 2014; 349: g6015.

124. Michaëlsson K, Wolk A, Langenskiöld S, Basu S, Lemming EW, Melhus H, Byberg L Milk intake and risk of mortality and fractures in women and men: cohort studies. BMJ; 2014; 349: g6015.

125. Kumar M, Kumar A, Nagpal R, Mohania D, Behare P, Verma V, Kumar P, Poddar D, Aggarwal PK, Henry CJ, Jain S, Yadav H. Cancer-preventing attributes of probiotics: an update. Int J Food Sci Nutr; 2010; 61: 473-96.

126. US Department of Commerce, US Census Bureau, The 2012 Statistical Abstract, report number 217 found at http://www.census.gov/compendia/statab/cats/health_nutrition/food_consumption_and_nutrition.html

127. American Heart Association, found at http://www.heart.org/HEARTORG/GettingHealthy/NutritionCenter/HealthyDietGoals/Sugars-and-Carbohydrates_UCM_303296_Article.jsp

128. University of Texas, SALSA study, found at http://www.uthscsa.edu/hscnews/singleformat2.asp?newID=3861

129. University of Texas, SALSA study, found at http://www.uthscsa.edu/hscnews/singleformat2.asp?newID=3861

130. Swithers S. Artificial sweeteners produce the counterintuitive effect of inducing metabolic derangements. Trends in Endocrinology and Metabolism, September 2013; 24 (9): 431–441.

131. Suez J, Korem T, Zeevi D, Zilberman-Schapira G, Thaiss CA, Maza O, Israeli D, Zmora N, Gilad S, Weiberger A, Kuperman Y, Harmelin A, Kolodkin I, Shapiro H, Halpern Z, Segal E, Elinav E. Artificial sweeteners induce glucose intolerance by altering the gut microbiota. Nature; October 2015, 514: 181–186.

132. Aris, A & Leblanc S. Maternal and fetal exposure to pesticides associated to genetically modified foods in Eastern Townships of Quebec. 2011 May; 31(4): 528-33.

133. Centers for Disease Control and Prevention (CDC). Investigation of human health effects associated with potential exposure to genetically modified corn. A report to the US Food and Drug Administration from the Centers for Disease Control and Prevention. National Center for Environmental Health; 2001.

CHAPTER 8:

134. Lee JH, Khor TO et al., Dietary Phytonutrients and Cancer Prevention: NRF2 signaling, epigenetics and cell death mechanisms in blocking cancer imitation and progression. Pharmacol Ther, Feb 2013; 137 (2): 153-171.

135. Johnson EJ. The role of carotenoids in human health. Nutr Clin Care, 2002 Mar-April; 5 (2): 56-65.

136. Giovannuccci E, Rimm EB et al., A prospective study of tomato products, lycopene and prostate cancer risk. J Natl Cancer Inst; 2002 Mar; 694(5): 391-8.

137. Karppi J, Laukkanen JA et al., Serum lycopene decreases the risk of stroke in men. Neurology, 2012 Oct; 79(15): 1540-47.

138. Johnson EJ. The role of carotenoids in human health. Nutr Clin Care, 2002; Mar-April; 5(2):56-65.

139. Hertog MG, Feskens EJ et al., Dietary antioxidants flavonoids and risk of coronary heart disease: the Zutphen Elderly Study. Lancet 1993; 342: 1007-1011.

140. Knekt P, Jarvinen R et al., Flavonoid intake and coronary mortality in Finland: a cohort study. BMJ, 1996; 312: 478-81.

141. Semba RD, Ferrucci L. et al., Reservatrol levels and all-cause mortality in older community-dwelling adults. JAMA Intern Med. 2014 July; (174(7): 1077-84

142. World Health Organization. Diet, nutrition, and the prevention of chronic diseases. Geneva: World Health Organization, 1990.

143. Joshipura KJ, Hu FB, Manson JE, et al., The effect of fruit and vegetable intake on risk for coronary heart disease. Ann Intern Med 2001; 134: 1106–14.

144. Leenders M, Sluijs I, Ros MM, et al., Fruit and vegetable consumption and mortality:European prospective investigation into cancer and nutrition. Am J Epidemiol 2013; 178: 590–602.

145. Oyebode O, Gordon-Dseagu V et al., Fruit and vegetable consumption and all-cause, cancer and CVD mortality: analysis of Health Survey for England data. J Epidemiol Community Health; Published Online First: 3/31/2014 doi:10.1136/jech-2013-203500

146. Dauchet L, Amouyel P, Hercberg S, et al., Fruit and vegetable consumption and risk of coronary heart disease: a meta-analysis of cohort studies. J Nutr 2006; 136: 2588–93.

147. Hu FB, Stampfer MJ et al., Dietary intake of alpha-linoleic acid and risk of ischemic heart disease among women. Am J Clin Nutr, 1999; 69: 890-7.

148. Liu S, Burin JE et al., A prospective study of dietary fiber intake and risk of cardio-vascular disease among women. JACC 2002; 39: 49-56.

149. Liu S, Stampfer MJ et al., Whole grain consumption and risk of coronary heart disease: results from the Nurses' Health Study. Am J Clin Nutr, 1999; 70: 412-419.

150. Berni Canini R, Di Costanzo M et al., Potential beneficial effects of butyrate in intestinal and extraintestinal diseases. World J Gastroenterol, Mar 28, 2011; 17(12): 1519–1528.

151. Ledikwe JH, Blanck HM, Kettel Khan L, et al., Dietary energy density is associated with energy intake and weight status in US adults. Am J Clin Nutr, 2006; 83: 1362-8.

152. Research to Practice Series No 5, Low-energy-dense foods and weight management: cutting calories while controlling hunger. National Center for Disease Control Prevention and Healthy Promotion.

153. Duncan KH, Bacon JA, Weinsier RL. The effects of high and low energy density diets on satiety, energy intake, and eating time of obese and nonobese subjects. American Journal of Clinical Nutrition, 1983; 37: 763-767

154. Shintani TT, Beckham S, Brown AC, O'Connor HK. The Hawaii Diet: ad libitum high carbohydrate, low fat multi-cultural diet for the reduction of chronic disease risk factors: obesity, hypertension, hypercholesterolemia, and hyperglycemia. Hawaii Medical Journal, 2001; 60: 69-73.

155. Ornish D, Schweritz LW et al., Intensive lifestyle changes for reversal of coronary heart disease. JAMA, December 16, 1998—Vol 280, No. 23

156. Kushi LH, Lenart EB et al., Health implications of Mediterranean diets in light of contemporary knowledge. 1. Plant foods and dairy products. Am J Clin Nutr, June 1995, 61: 1407S-1415S

157. Hu FB, Williett WC. Optimal diets for prevention of coronary heart disease.disease. JAMA; 2002Nov 27; 288(20): 2569-78.

158. de Lorgeril M, Renaud S, Mamelle N, et al., Mediterranean alpha-linolenic acid-rich diet in secondary prevention of coronary heart disease. Lancet, 1994; 343: 1454–9

159. Appel L, Moore TJ, Obrazanek E, for the DASH Collaborative Research Group. A clinical trial of the effects of dietary patterns on blood pressure. N Engl J Med, 1997; 336: 1117–24

160. Jacobs DR Jr, Meyer KA, Kushi LH, Folsom AR. Whole-grain intake may reduce the risk of ischemic heart disease death in postmenopausal women: the Iowa Women's Health Study. Am J Clin Nutr, 1998; 68: 248–57.

161. Liu S, Stampfer MJ, Hu FB, et al., Whole-grain consumption and risk of coronary heart disease: results from the Nurses' Health Study. Am J Clin Nutr, 1999; 70: 412–9

162. Fung TT, Willett WC, Stampfer MJ, Manson JE, Hu FB. Dietary patterns and risk of coronary heart disease in women. Arch Intern Med 2001; 161: 1857–62

163. Hu FB, Rimm EB, Stampfer MJ, Ascherio A, Spiegelman D, Willett WC. Prospective study of major dietary patterns and risk of coronary heart disease in men. Am J Clin Nutr, 2000; 72: 912–21

164. Crous-Bou M, Fung TT, Prescott J, Julin B, Du M, Sun Q, Rexode KM, Hu FB, De Vivo I, Mediterranean diet and telomere length in Nurses' Health Study: population based cohort study, BMJ, Dec 2014, 349

165. Mann, Traci; Tomiyama, A. Janet; Westling, Erika; Lew, Ann-Marie; Samuels, Barbra; Chatman, Jason. American Psychologist, Vol 62(3), Apr 2007; 220-233

166. National Institute of Diabetes and Digestive and Kidney Disease, Weight Control Information Network, found at http://win.niddk.nih.gov/publications/myths. htm

CHAPTER 9:

167. Anitschkov NN. A history of experimentation on arterial atherosclerosis in animals. In: Bleumenthal HT ed. Cowdry's Arteriosclerosis: A Survey of the Problem. 2nd ed. Springfield Ill: Charles C Thomas; 1967: 21-44.

168. McGill HC. The relationship of dietary cholesterol to serum cholesterol concentration and to atherosclerosis in man. Am J Clin Nutr, 1979; 32: 2664-2702.

169. Hu FB, Willett WC. Optimal diets for prevention of coronary heart disease. Clinical Cardiology, JAMA, 2002; 288(20): 22569-2578.

170. Gordon T: The diet-heart idea: outline of a history. Am J Epidemiol, 1988; 127: 220-225.

171. Keys A. Coronary heart disease in seven countries. Circulation (Suppl I), 41-42: 1-211.

172. Kang JX, Leaf A. Antiarrhythmic effects of polyunsaturated fatty acids: recent studies. Circulation,1996; 94: 1774-1780

173. Connor SL, Connor WE. Are fish oils beneficial in the prevention and treatment of coronary artery disease? Am J Clin Nutr, 1997; 66(4 suppl): 1020S-1031S

174. Kromhout D, Bosscheiter EB, de Lezenne Coulander C. The inverse relation between fish consumption and 20-year mortality from coronary heart disease. N Engl J Med,1985; 312: 1205-1209

175. Hu FB, Willett WC. Optimal diets for prevention of coronary heart disease. Clinical Cardiology, JAMA, 2002; 288(20): 22569-2578

176. Pietinen P, Ascherio A, Korhonen P. et al., Intake of fatty acids and risk of coronary heart disease in a cohort of Finnish men: the ATBC Study. Am J Epidemiol, 1997; 145: 876-887

177. Ascherio A, Rimm EB, Giovannucci EL, Spiegelman D, Stampfer MJ, Willett WC. Dietary fat and risk of coronary heart disease in men: cohort follow-up study in the United States. BMJ, 1996; 313: 84-90

178. Steinberg D, Parthasarathy S, Carew TE, Khoo JC, Witztum JL. Beyond cholesterol: modifications of low-density lipoprotein that increase its atherogenicity. N Engl J Med, 1989; 320: 915–924

179. Mozaffarian D, Rimm EB, Herrington DM. Dietary fats, carbohydrate, and progression of coronary atherosclerosis in postmenopausal women. Am J Clin Nutr, 2004; 80: 1175–1184

180. Mensink RP, Katan MB. Effect of dietary fatty acids on serum lipids and lipoproteins: a meta-analysis of 27 trials. Arterioscler Thromb, 1992; 12: 911–919

181. Harris WS, Mozaffariann D et al., Omega-6 fatty acids and risk for cardiovascular disease. Circulation, 2009; 119: 902-907

182. Laaksonen DE, Nyyssonen K, Niskanen L, Rissanen TH, Salonen JT. Prediction of cardiovascular mortality in middle-aged men by dietary and serum linoleic and polyunsaturated fatty acids. Arch Intern Med. 2005; 165: 193–199

183. Harris WS, Mozaffariann D et al., Omega-6 fatty acids and risk for cardiovascular disease. Circulation, 2009; 119: 902-907

184. http://www.umm.edu/altmed/articles/omega-6-000317.htm

185. Mensink RP, Katan MB. Effect of dietary trans fatty acids on high-density and low-density lipoprotein cholesterols levels in healthy subects. NEJM, 1990; 323: 439-445.

186. Nestel P, Noakes M et al., Plasma lipoprotein and Lp [a] changes with substitution of eladic acid for oleic acid in the diet. J Lipi Res, 1992; 33: 1029-1036.

187. Katan MB, Zock PL. Trans fatty acids and their effects on lipoproteins in humans. Annu Rev Nutr,1995; 15: 473-493.

188. Salmeron J, Hu FB, Manson JE et al., Dietary fat intake and risk of type 2 diabetes in women. Am J Clin Nutr, 2001; 73: 1019-1026

189. Kushi LH, Lew RA, Stare FJ. et al., Diet and 20-year mortality from coronary heart disease: the Ireland-Boston Diet-Heart Study, N Engl J Med,1985; 312: 811-818

190. Hu FB, Stampfer MJ, Manson JE et al., Dietary fat intake and the risk of coronary heart disease in women. N Engl J Med, 1997; 337: 1491-1499

191. Estruch R, Ros E et al., Primary prevention of cardiovascular disease with a Mediterranean diet. NEJM, April 2013; 368: 14; 1279-90.

192. Kris-Etherton PM for the Nutrition Committee. Circulation;1999;100: 1253-58

193. Rudel L, Parks J et al., Compared with dietary monounsaturated and saturated fat, polyunsaturated fat protects African green monkeys from coronary artery atherosclerosis. Arteriosclerosis, Thrombosis, and Vascular Biology, 1995; 15: 2101-2110 doi: 10.1161/01.ATV.15.12.2101

194. Novick J. https://www.pritikin.com/your-health/healthy-living/eating-right/1103-whats-wrong-with-olive-oil.html#.VF5MF_J0yP8

195. Vogel R, Coretti M et al., The postprandial effect of components of the Mediterranean diet on endothelial function. J Am Coll Card, 2000; 36: 1455.

196. Trichopoulou A, Barnia C et al., Anatomy of health effects of Mediterranean diet: Greek EPIC prospective cohort study. BMJ, 2009; 338: b2337

197. Hopkins P. Effects of dietary cholesterol on serum cholesterol: a meta-analysis and review. Am J Clin Nutr, June 1992;55(6):1060-1070 6 1060-1070

198. Chowdury R, Warnakula S et al., Association of dietary, circulating, and supplement fatty acids with coronary risk: a systematic review and meta-analysis. Ann Intern Med,2014; 160(6): 398-406 (ISSN: 1539-3704)

199. Assunção ML, Ferreira HS et al., Effects of dietary coconut oil on the biochemical and anthropometric profiles of women presenting abdominal obesity. Lipids, Format··See comment in PubMed Commons belo2009 Jul; 44(7): 593-601. doi: 10.1007/s11745-009-3306-6. Epub 2009 May 13.

200. Barry Em, Eisenberger S et al., Effects of diets rich in monounsaturated fatty acids on plasma lipoproteins—the Jerusalem Nutrition Study. II. Monounsaturated fatty acids vs carbohydrates. Am J Clin Nutr,,1992 Aug; 56(2): 394-403.

201. Ros E, Nunez I et al., A walnut diet improves endothelial function in hypercholesterolemic subjects. Circulation, 2004; 109: 1609-1614

202. Fraser G, Sabate J et al., A possible protective effect of nut consumption on risk of coronary heart disease: : The Adventist Health Study. Arch Intern Med, 1992; 152(7): 1416-1424. doi:10.1001/archinte.1992.00400190054010

203. Sabate J, Fraser GE et al., Effects of walnuts on serum lipid levels and blood pressure in normal med. NEJM, 3/1993; 329)9): 603-7

204. Hu F, Stampfer M et al., Frequent nut consumption and risk of coronary heart disease in women: prospective cohort study. BMJ, 1998; 317: 1341

205. Sabate J, Oda K et al., Nut consumption and blood lipid levels: : A Pooled Analysis of 25 Intervention Trials. Arch Intern Med, 2010; 170(9): 821-827. doi:10.1001/archinternmed.2010.79.

206. Ros E, Nunez I et al., A walnut diet improves endothelial function in hypercholesterolemic subjects. Circulation, 2004; 109: 1609-1614

207. Alpher CM, Mattes RD. Peanut consumption improves indices of cardiovascular disease risk in healthy adults. J Am Clin Nutr, 22: 2; 2003

208. Jenkins D, Kendall C et al., Dose response of almonds on coronary heart disease risk factors: blood lipids, oxidized low-density lipoproteins, lipoprotein(a), homocysteine, and pulmonary nitric oxide. Circulation. 2002; 106: 1327-1332

209. Zatónski W, Campos H, Willett W. Rapid declines in coronary heart disease mortality in Eastern Europe are associated with increased consumption of oils rich in alpha-linolenic acid. Eur J Epidemiol, 2008; 23: 3–10. doi: 10.1007/s10654-007-9195-1.

210. Campos H, Baylin A, Willett WC. Alpha-linolenic acid and risk of nonfatal acute myocardial infarction. Circulation, 2008; 118: 339–345. doi: 10.1161/CIRCULATIONAHA.107.762419

CHAPTER 10:

211. Sanchez E, Kelley KM. Herb and Spice History. Penn State College of Agricultural Sciences, Department of Horticulture, http://extension.psu.edu/plants/gardening/fact-sheets/herbs/herb-and-spice-history/extension_publication_file

212. Aggarwal B, Yost D. Healing Spices: How to Use 50 Everyday and Exotic Spices to Boost Health and Beat Disease. Jan 2011.

213. Kuptniratsaikul V, Dajpratham P et al., Efficacy and safety of curcuma domestica extracts compared with ibuprofen in patients with knee osteoarthritis: a multicenter study. Clin Interv Aging, 2014; 9: 451-8. Epub 2014 Mar 20. PMID: 24672232

214. Aggarwal B, Yost D. Healing Spices: How to Use 50 Everyday and Exotic Spices to Boost Health and Beat Disease. Jan 2011.

215. Fratiglioni L, De Ronchi D, Agüero-Torres H, Worldwide prevalence and incidence of dementia. Drugs Aging, 1999 Nov; 15(5):365-75.

216. Yang F, Lim GP, Begum AN, Ubeda OJ, Simmons MR, Ambegaokar SS, Chen PP, Kayed R, Glabe CG, Frautschy SA, Cole GM, Curcumin inhibits formation of amyloid beta oligomers and fibrils, binds plaques, and reduces amyloid in vivo. J Biol Chem. 2005 Feb 18; 280(7):5892-901.

217. Aggarwal B, Yost D. Healing Spices: How to Use 50 Everyday and Exotic Spices to Boost Health and Beat Disease. Jan 2011.

218. Min Y, Kwang HH, et al., Curcumin attenuates adhesion molecules and matrix metalloproteinase expression in hypercholesterolemic rabbits. Nutrition Research, Volume 34, Issue 10, October 2014; pp 886-893

219. Puangsombat K, Smith JS. Inhibition of heterocyclic amine formation in beef patties by ethanolic extracts of rosemary. See comment in PubMed Commons below] Food Sci., 2010 Mar;75(2): T40-7. doi: 10.1111/j.1750-3841.2009.01491.x.

220. Khan A, SafdarM et al., Cinnamon improves glucose and lipids of people with type 2 diabetes. 10.2337/diacare.26.12.3215 Diabetes Care December 2003; vol. 26 no. 12 3215-3218

221. Couturier K, Batandier C. Cinnamon improves insulin sensitivity and alters the body composition in an animal ,odel of the metabolic syndrome., 2010 Sep 1; 501(1): 158-61. doi: 10.1016/j.abb.2010.05.032. Epub 2010 May 31.

222. Cheng SS, Liu JY et al., Chemical polymorphism and antifungal activity of essential oils from leaves of different provenances of indigenous cinnamon., January 2006: pp 306–312

223. Rosti L, Gastaldi G, Frigiola A. Cinnamon and bacterial enteric infections. Ind J Ped 2008, 75: 529-530

224. Zhu M, Carvalho R, Scher A, Wu CD. Short-term germ-killing effect of sugar-sweetened cinnamon chewing gum on salivary anaerobes associated with halitosis. J Clin Dent 2011, 22: 23-26

225. Jayaprakasha GK, Jagan Mohan Rao L, Sakariah KK: Volatile constituents from cinnamomum zeylanicum fruit stalks and their antioxidant activities. J Agric Food Chem 2003; 51: 4344-4348.

226. Rahman K, Lowe GM. Garlic and cardiovascular disease: a critical review. J Nutr, March 2006;136(3):736S-740S

227. Stevinson C, Pittler MH, Ernst E. Garlic for treating hypercholesterolemia. a meta-analysis of randomised clinical trials. Ann Intern Med, 2000;19: 420–9

228. Rahman K, Lowe GM. Garlic and cardiovascular disease: a critical review, J Nutr; March 2006 vol. 136 no. 3: 736S-740S

229. Breithaupt-Grogler K, Ling M, Boudoulas H, Belz GG, Heiden M, Wenzel E, Gu LD. Protective effect of chronic garlic intake on elastic properties of aorta in the elderly. Circulation, 1997; 96: 2649–55

CHAPTER 11

230. Askew EW, University of Utah, healthcare.utah.edu/publicaffairs/news

CHAPTER 12:

231. Sleep at the Wheel: the prevalence and impact of drowsy driving. AAA Foundation for traffic safety, November 2010.

232. Hirshkowitz M, Whiton K, Albert S M, et al., National Sleep Foundation 's sleep time duration recommendations: methodology and results summary. 2015 Jan,

233. Spiegel K, Leproult R, Van Cauter E. Impact of sleep debt on metabolic and endocrine function. Lancet. 1999; 354: 1435-1439

234. Sleep foundation. www.sleepfoundation.org

235. Spiegel K, Leproult R, Van CauterE. Impact of sleep debt on metabolic and endocrine function . Lancet, Oct 23, 1999; 354(9188): 1435-9.

236. Speigel K, Leproult R, Van Cauter E. Impact of sleep debt on metabolic and endocrine function. Lancet, Oct 1999; 354 (9188):1435-9.

237. Vgontzas AN, Zoumakis E, et al., Adverse effects of modest sleep restriction on sleepiness,performance, and inflammatory cytokines. J CLin Endocrinol Metab. 2004; 89(5): 2119

238. Tsai K, Hsu TG, LuFJ, Hsu CF, Lu FJ,, and Kong CW. Age–related changes in the mitochondrial depolarization induced by oxidative injury in human peripheral blood leukocytes. Free Radic Res, 2001; 35: 251-255

239. Yang S, Porter VA, et al., Effects of oxidant stress on inflammation and survival of iNOS knockout mice after marrow transplantation. AM J Physiol Lung Cell Mol Physiology, 2001; 281: 922-L930

240. Everson C, Laatsch CD, Neil H. Antioxidant defense responses to sleep loss and sleep recovery. Am J Phsiol Regul Integr Comp Physiol, 2005; 288: R374-383

241. Liebler DC, Reed DJ. Free-radical defense and repair mechanisms . Free radical Toxicology, edited by Wallace KB. Washington , DC: Tayler & Francis. 1997; p141-171

242. Everson CA, Laatsch CD, Hogg N. Antioxidant defense responses to sleep loss and recovery. American Journal of Physiology, 2005;288 (2):R374-383.

243. Droge W, Breitkreutz R. Glutathione and immune function. Proc Nutr Soc., Nov 2000; 59(4): 595-600.

244. Summala H, Mikkota Hum Factors. Fatal accidents among car and truck drivers: effects of fatigue. age, and alcohol consumption. From up to date definition and consequences of sleep deprivation, 1994; 36(2): 315

245. Van Dongen HP, Maislin G, Mullington JM, Dinges DF. The cumulative cost of additional wakefulness: dose–response effects on neurobehavioral functions and sleep physiology from chronic sleep restriction and total sleep deprivation. Sleep, 2003; 26(2): 117

246. Jones M. How little sleep get you get away with? New York Times Magazine, April 15,2011; (margueritepjones@gmail.com)

247. Goel N, Rao H, Durmer JS, Dinges DF. Neurocognitive Consequences of Sleep Deprivation. Semin Neurol, 2009: 29(4):320-339.

248. Bonnet MH, Arand DL. We are chronically sleep deprived. Sleep, 1995; 18(10): 908

249. Van Cauter E, Polonsky KS et al., Roles of circadian rhythmicity and sleep in human glucose regulation. Endocr Rev.,1997; 18(5): 716–738.

250. Taheri S, Lin L, Austin D, Young T, Mignot E. Short sleep duration is associated with reduced leptin, elevated ghrelin, and increased body mass index. PLoS Med, 2004; 1(3):e62.

251. Scott EM, Carter AM, Grant PJ. Association between polymorphisms in the clock gene, obesity and the metabolic syndrome in man. Int J Obes (Lond), 2008; 32(4): 658–662.

252. Gangwisch J, Heymsfield S, Boden-Albala B , et al. Sleep Duration as a Risk Factor for Diabetes Incidence in a Large US Sample. Sleep, 2007 ; 30 (12):1667-1673

253. Knutson RL. Impact of sleep and sleep loss on glucose homeostasis and appetite regulation. Sleep Med Clinic. June 2007; 2(2):187-197.

254. Engle-Friedman M. The effects of sleep loss on capacity and effort . Sleep Science (2014), http://dx.doi.org/10.

255. Insomnia with short sleep duration and mortality: the Penn State cohort. Vgontzaz AN, Liao D. Pejovic S et al. Sleep, 2010; 33(9):1159.

256. Sleep disorders and sleep deprivation: an unmet public health problem, Consensus Report. March 2006. Biomedical and Health Research, Institute of Medicine of the National Academies

257. Taheri S, Lin L, Austin D, Young T, Mignot E. Short sleep duration is associated with reduced leptin, elevated ghrelin, and increased body mass index. PLoS Med, 2004; 1(3):e62.

258. Nedeltcheva AV, Kilkus JM, Imperial J, Schoeller DA, Penev PD. Insufficient sleep undermines dietary efforts to reduce adiposity. Annals of Internal Medicine, 2010 ;153(7): 435-441.

259. Prince TM, Abel T. The Impact of Sleep Loss on Hippocampal Function. Learning and Memory. 2013, 20:558-569

260. Gais S, Born J. Declarative memory consolidation: Mechanisms acting during human sleep, Learning and Memory, 2004, 11: 679-685

261. Payne JD, Nadel L. Sleep, dreams, and memory consolidation: The role of the stress hormone cortisol. Learn Mem, Nov 2004; 11(6): 671-678.

262. Kumar R1, Birrer BV et al. Reduced mammillary body volume in patients with obstructive sleep apnea. Neuroscience Lett, 2008 June 27; 438(3): 330-334

263. Kato M, Roberts-Thompson P, Philips BG, et al., Impairment of endothelium–dependent vasodilation of resistance vessels in patients with obstructive sleep apnea. Circulation, 200; 102: 2607-2610.

264. Kumar R, Birrer BV, Macey PM, Woo MA, Gupta RK, Yan-Go FL, Harper RM. Reduced mammillary body volume in patients with obstructive sleep apnea. Neuroscience Lett, 2008 June 27; 438(3): 330-334

265. Srinivasan V, Pandi-Perumal SR, Brzeinski A, Bhatnagar KP, Cardinalli OP. Melatonin Immune fuction and cancer. Recent Pat Endocr Metab Immune Drug Diseases, 2011 May;5(2):107-23.

266. Blask De. Melatonin, sleep disturbance and cancer risk. Sleep Medicine Reviews, 2009; 257-264

267. Hansen J. Increased breast cancer risk among women who work predominantly at night. Epidemilogy, 2001; (12): 74-77

268. Feychting M ,Osterlund B, Ahlbom A. Reduced cancer incidence among the blind. Epidemiology. 1998; (9): 490-494

269. Chang AM, Aeschbach D, Duffy JF. Evening use of light –emitting eReaders negatively affects sleep, circadian timing, and next –morning alertness. PNAS 2015; 112 (4); 1232-1237

270. Ackermann K, Bux Roman, Rub Udo, et al., Melatonin synthesis in the human pineal gland. BMC Neuroscience. 2007 Mar,8 (1): P2.

271. Cajochen C, Munch M, Kobialka S, Krauchi K, Steiner R, Oelhafen P, Orgul S, Wirz-Justice A:High sensitivity of human melatonin, alertness, thermoregulation and heart rate to short wavelength light. J Clin Endo Met ,2005; 90: 1311-1316.

272. Figueiro MG, Bierman A, Plitnick B, et al. Preliminary evidence that both blue and red light can induce alertness at night. BMC Neuroscience, 2009; 10: 105.

273. Figueiro MG, Bierman A, Plitnick B, et al. Preliminary evidence that both blue and red light can induce alertness at night. BMC Neuroscience, 2009; 10: 105.

274. Dahl R E, Lewin D S. Pathways to adolescent health sleep regulation and behavior. Journal of Adolescent Health, 2002; 31 (6); 175-184

275. Oakley , Barbara M. A mind for numbers. New York: Penguin Group. 2014. Print.

CHAPTER 13:

276. Sengupta Health Impacts of Yoga and Pranayama: a state–of–the–art review. Int J Prev Med, Jul 2012; 3 (7): 444-458

277. Yogananda. Autobiography of a yogi. Los Angeles, California: Self Realization Fellowship. 2006 .Print

278. Gothe NP, Kramer AF, McAuley E. The effects of an 8 week Hatha yoga intervention on executive function in older adults. J Gerontol A Biol Sci Med Sci, 2014 Sep ; 69(9): 1109-16

279. Crow EM, Jeannot E, Trewhela A. Effectiveness of Iyengar yoga in treating spinal (back and neck) pain: a systematic review. Int J Yoga, 2015; 8(1): 3-14

280. Udupa K, Madanmohan, Bhavanani AB et al., Effect of pranayama training on cardiac function in normal young volunteers. Indian J Physiolo Pharmacol, Jan 2003; 41(1): 27-33

281. Kaswal D, Shah Shamik, Mishra Avantika et al., Can yoga be used to treat gastro-esophageal reflux diease? 2013 July-Dec; 6(2): 131-133

282. Ricard M, Lutz A, Davidson R. Mind of the meditator. Scientific American, 2014: 39-45.

283. Ricard M, Lutz A, Davidson R. Mind of the meditator. Scientific American, 2014: 39-45

284. Lazar, SW, Kerr CE, Wasserman RU, et al., Meditation experience is associated with increased cortical thickness. Neuroreport, 2006 Nov; 16 (17): 1893-7.

285. Gottselig JM, Hofer-Tinguely G, Borbely AA, et al., Sleep and rest facilitate auditory learning. Neurosci, 2004; 127: 557-561.

286. Lazar, SW, Kerr CE, Wasserman RU, et al., Meditation experience is associated with increased cortical thickness. Neuroreport, 2006 Nov; 16 (17): 1893-7.

287. Dangwal, Parmesh. "I Dare!": Kiran Bedi:N.p,:Sangam, 2001. Print.

288. Brewington K. Yoga, meditation program helps city youth cope with stress. The Baltimore Sun Feb 2011: n. 2011. Print

289. Sullivan B, Thompson H. "Brain, Interrupted," The New York Times 2013: n. page. Print

290. Creswell JD, Irwin MR, Burklund LJ. Mindfulness–based stress reduction training reduces loneliness and pro–inflammatory gene expression in older adults: a small randomized controlled trial. Brain Behav Immun, 2012 Oct; 26 (7): 1095-101.

291. Banaski J, Williams H, Haberman M. Effect of Iyengar yoga practice on fatigue and diurnal salivary cortisol concentration in breast cancer survivors. J Am Acad Nurse Pract, 2011 Mar; 23(3): 135-42

292. Yadav RK, Magan D, Mehta N. Efficacy of a short- term yoga-based lifestyle intervention in reducing stress and inflammation: preliminary results. J Altern Complement Med, 2012 Jul; 18(7): 662-667

293. Thirthalli J, Naveen GH, Rao MG. Cortisol and antidepressant effects of yoga. Indian J Psychiatry, 2013 Jul; 55(3): S405- 408.

294. Banasik J, Williams H, Haberman M, Blank SE, Bendel R, Effect of Iyengar yoga practice on fatigue and diurnal salivary cortisol concentration in breast cancer survivors. J AM Acad Nurse Pract, 2011 Mar; 23(3): 135-42.

295. Black DS, Cole SW, Irwin MR, Breen E, St Cyr NM, Nazarian N, Khalsa DS, Lavretsky H. Yogic meditation reverses NF-KB and IRF–related transcriptome dynamics in leukocytes of family dementia caregvers in a randomized controlled trial. Psychoneuroendocrinology, 2013 Mar; 38(3): 348-55.

296. Black DS, Cole SW, Irwin MR, Breen E, St Cyr NM, Nazarian N, Khalsa DS, Lavretsky H. Yogic meditation reverses NF-KB and IRF related transcriptome dynamics of leukocytes of family dementia caregivers in a randomized controlled trial. Psychoneuroendocrinolgy. 2013 Mar; 38(3): 348-55.

297. Chatterjee S, Mondal S. Effect of regular yogic training on growth hormone and dehydroepiandrosterone sulfate as an endocrine marker of aging. Evidence Based Complementary and Alternative Medicine, 2014

298. Sarvottam K, Magan D, Yadav RK, Mehta N, Mahapatra SC. Adiponectin, interleukin -6 and cardiovascular disease risk factors are modified by a short–term yoga–based lifestyle intervention in overweight and obese men. J Alter Complement Med, 2013 May; 19(5): 397-402.

299. Nidhi R, Padmalatha V, Nagarathna R. Effect of a yoga program on glucose metabolism and blood lipid levels in adolescent girls with polycystic ovary syndrome. Int J Gynaecol Obstet, 2012 Jul; 118 (1): 37- 41

300. Sengupta, P. Health impacts of yoga and pranayama: a state-of-the-art review. Int J Prev Med, 2012 Jul; 3(7); 444-458.

301. Ghiadone L, Donald AE, Cropley M, Mullen MJ, Oakely G, Taylor M, O'Conner G, Betteridge J, Klein N, Steptoe A, Deanfield JE. Mental stress induces transient endothelial dysfunction in humans. Clinical Investigation and Reports. Circulation., 2000; 102: 2473-2478.

302. Sivasankara S, Pollard-Quintner S, Sachdeva PR, Pugeda J, Hoq SM, Zarich SW. The effect of a six week program of yoga and meditation on brachial artery reactivity. Do psycholoscoial interventionsl affect tones. Clin Clin Cardiolo, 2006; 29: 393-398.

303. Ornish D, Scherwitz LW, Doody RS. Effects of stress management training and dietary changes in treating ischemic heart disease. JAMA, 1983 Jan; 249(1): 54-59.

304. Cramer H, Lauch R, Haller H, Dobos G, Michalsen A. et al., A systematic review of yoga for heart disease. European Journal of Preventive Cardiology, 2015 Mar: 22(3): 284-295.

305. Zernicke KA, Campbell TS, Blustein PK. Mindfulness–based stress reduction for the treatment of irritable bowel syndrome symptoms: a randomized wait –list controlled trial . Int J Behav Med, 2013 Sept; 20 (3) :385-96

306. Goyal M, Singh S, Sibinga EMS. Meditation Programs for Psychological stress and Well-being. A Systematic Review and Meta –analysis. JAMA, 2014; 174 (3) : 357-468.

307. Jedel S, Hoffman A, Meriman P. A randomized controlled trial of mindfulness–based stress reduction to prevent flare-ups in patients with inactive ulcerative colitis. Digestion, 2014; 89(2): 142-55

308. Singh, G, Singh J. Yoga Nidra: a deep mental relaxation approach . Br J Sports Med. 2010; 44: i71-i72.

309. Walton KG., et al., Lowering cortisol and CVD risk in postmenopausal women: a pilot study using the Transccendental Meditation program. Annals of New York Academy of Sciences. 2005; 1032: 211-215

310. Schneider RH. Altered responses of cortisol, GH, TSH and testosterone to acute stress after four months' practice of Transcendental Meditation . Annals of the New York Academy of Sciences, 1994; 746: 381-384.

311. Ray Indranill Basu, Menezes AR, Malur AR, et al., Meditation and coronary heart disease: a review of the current clinical evidence. The Ochsner Journal, 2014; 14: 696-703.

312. Schneider RH, Grim CE, Rainforth MV, Kotchen T, Nidich SI, Gaylord-King C, Salerno JW, Kotchen JM, Alexander CN. Stress reduction in the secondary prevention of cardiovascular disease: randomized controlled trial of Transcendental Meditation and health education in Blacks. Circulation: Cardiovascular Quality and Outcomes, 2012; 5: 750-758.

313. Brook, R D, Appel LJ, Rajagopalan S. AHA Scientfic Statement. Beyond medications and diet: alternative apporaches to lowering blood pressure. A scientific statement from the AHA. Hypertension. 2013

314. Liu XC, Pan L, Hu Q, Donq WP, Yan JH, Donq L. Effects of yoga training in patients with chronic obstructive pulmonary disease: a systematic reiew and meta-anlaysis. J Thorac Dis, 2014 Jun; 6(6): 795-802.

315. Berkowitz B, Clark P . The health hazards of sitting. Washington Post. Jan 2014

316. Singh S, Kylzom T, Singh KP, Tandon OP, Madhu SV. Influence of pranayamas and yoga – asanas on serum insulin, blood glucose and lipid profile in type 2 diabetes. Indian Journal of Clinical Biochemistry, 2008; 22(4): 365-368.

317. Manjunatha S, Vempati RP, Ghosh D, Bijlani RL. An investigation into the acute and long–term effects of selected yogic postures on fasting and post prandial glycemia and insulinemia in healthy young subjects. Indian J Physiol Pharmacol, 2005; Jul-Sept: 49: (3): 319-24

318. Bhasin MK, Dusek JA, Chang E-H, Joseph MG, Denninger JW, Fricchione GL, Benson H, Libermann TA. Relaxation response induces temporal transcriptome changes In energy metabolism, insulin secretion and inflammatory pathways. PLOS One.2013 May

319. Bhasin MK, Dusek JA, Chang E-H, Joseph MG, Denninger JW, Fricchione GL, Benson H, Libermann TA. Relaxation response induces temporal transcriptome changes In energy metabolism, insulin secretion and inflammatory pathways. PLOS One. 2013, May

CHAPTER 14:

320. Puetz TW. Physical activity and feelings of energy and fatigue: epidemiological evidence Sports Med, 2006; 36(9): 767-80

321. Conn VS, Hafdahl AR, Brown LM. Meta-analysis of quality of life outcomes from physical activity interventions. Nurs Res, 2009; 58(3): 175-83.

322. Conn VS, Hafdahl AR, Brown LM. Meta–analysis of quality of life outcomes from physical activity interventions. Nurs Res, 2009; 58(3): 175-83.

323. Garber CE, Blissmer B, Deschenes MR et al., Quantity and quality of exercise for developing and maintaining cardiorespiratory, musculoskeletal, and neuromotor fitness in apparently healthy adults: guidance for prescribing exercise. Medicine & Science in Sports and Exercise, 2011; DOI :10.1249/MSS.0b013e318213fefb.

324. Haskell WL, Lee I-M, Pate RR, Powell KE, Blair SN, Franklin BA, Macera CA, Heath GW, Thompson PD, Bauman A. Physical activity and public health: updated recommendations for adults from the American College of Sports Medicine and the American Heart Association. Circulation, 2007; 116 (9):1081-1093.

325. General Physical Activities Defined by Level of Intensity

326. Lee IM, Rexrode KM, Cook NR, Manson JE, Buring JE. Physical activity and coronary heart disease in women:is "no pain , no gain"passe? JAMA .2001; 285(11): 1447-54.

327. Manson, JE, Greenland P, LaCroix AZ, Stenfanick ML, Mouton CP, Oberman A, Perri MG, Sheps DS, Pettinger MB, Sicovick DS, Manson JE, Greenland P, LaCroix AZ Walking compared with vigorous exercise for the prevention of cardiovascular events in women. N Engl J Med, 2002; 347: 716-25.

328. Seeso HD, Paffenbarger RS Jr. , Lee IM. Physical activity and coronary heart disease in men: the Harvard Alumni Health Study. Circulation, 2000; 102(9): 975-80.

329. Tanasescu M, Leitzmann MF, Rimm EB,Willett WC, Stampfer MJ, Hu FB. Exercise type and intensity in relation to coronary heart disease in men. JAMA, 2002: 288(16): 1994-2000.

330. US Department of Health and Human Services. 2008 Physical Activity Guidelines for Americans [Internet]. Washington (DC): ODPHP Publication No. UU0036.2008 [cited 2010 Oct 10]. 61p.

331. Healy GN, Dustan DQ, Salmon J, Cerin E, Shaw JE, Zimmet PZ, Owen N. Breaks in Sedentary Time: Beneficial Associations with Metabolic Risk, Diabetes Care, April 2008; 31: 661-6.

332. 2014 Annual Report. America's Health Rankings. United Health Foundation. Americashealthrankings.org. Jan 2015.

333. Warren TY, Barry V, Hooker SP, Sui X, Church TS, Blair SN. Sedentary behaviors increase risk of cardiovascular disease mortality in men. Med Sci Sports Exerc, 2010; 42(5): 879-85.

334. Teychenne M, Ball K, Salmon J. Sedentary behavior and depression among adults: a review. Int J Behav Med, 2010; 17(4): 246-54.

335. Healy GN, Dustan DQ, Salmon J, Shaw JE, Zimmet PZ, Owen N. Television time and continuous metabolic risk in physically active adults. Med Sci Sports Exerc, 2008; 40 (4): 639-45.

336. US Department of Health and Human Services. Physical Activity Guidelines Advisory Committee Report, 2008[Internet]. Washington (DC): ODPHP Publication No. U0049. 2008[cited 2010 Sep 24]. 683p. Available from: http://www.health.gov/paguidelines/Report/pdf/CommitteeReport.pdf.

337. Whaley MH. (2006) ACSM'S Guidelines For Exercise Testing And Prescription Seventh Edition. Baltimore, Maryland: Lippincott Williams & Wilkins.

338. Bravata DM, Smith-Spangler C, Sundaram V,Gienger AL, Lin N, Lewis R, Stave CD, Olkin I, Sirard JR. Using pedometers to increase physical activity and improve health: a systematic review. JAMA,.2007; 298(19): 2296-304.

339. Kang M, Marshall SJ, Barreira TV, Lee JO. Effect of pedometer-based physical activity interventions: a meta –analysis. Res Q Exer Sport, 2009: 80 (3): 648-55.

340. Butcher LR, Thomas A, Backx K, Roberts AW, Morris K. Low–intensity exercise exerts beneficial effects on plasma lipids via PPAR gamma. Med Sci Sports Exerc. 2008; 40(7): 1263-70.

341. Bravata DM, Smith-Spangler C, Sundaram V, V,Gienger AL, Lin N, Lewis R, Stave CD, Olkin I, Sirard JR. Using pedometers to increase physical activity and improve health: a systematic review. JAMA, 2007; 298(19): 2296-304.

342. Bravata DM, Smith-Spangler C, Sundaram V, V,Gienger AL, Lin N, Lewis R, Stave CD, Olkin I, Sirard JR. Using pedometers to increase physical activity and improve health: a systematic review. JAMA, 2007; 298(19): 2296-304.

343. Owen N, Healy GN, Matthews CE, Dunstan QW, Too Much Sitting: Population-Health Science of Sedentary Behavior, Exerc Sports Sci Rev, July 2010; 35: 105-113.

344. Source from mayoclinic.org

345. Source from mayoclinic.org

346. Boreham , C. The Physiology of Training. UK: Elsevier Limited, 2006. Print.

347. Sulerman, Amer, and Craig C . Young. "Exercise Physiology." Medscape. N.p.,13 July 2013. Web. 10 Sept.2014.

348. Jenkins NT, Witkowski S, Spangenburg EE, Hagberg JM. Effects of acute and chronic endurance exercise on intracellular nitric oxide in putative endothelial progenitor cells: role of NAPDH oxidase. Am J Physiol Heart Circ Physiol, 2009 Nov; 297(5): 798-805.

349. McAllister RM, Newcomer SC, Laughlin H. Vascular nitric oxide: effects of exercise training in animals. Applied Physiology, Nutrition, and Metabolism, 2008; 33 (1): 173-178.

350. Jungersten L, Ambring A, Wall B, Wennmalm A. Both physical fitness and acute exercise regulate nitric oxide formation in healthy humans. J Appl Physiol, 1997; 82: 760-764.

351. De Fransceshi MS, Palange AL, Mancuso A, Grande L, Muccari D, Scavelli FB, Irace C, Gnasso A, Carallo C. Decreased platelet aggregation by sheer stress-stimulated endothelial cells in vitro: description of a method and first results in diabetes. Diab Vasc Dis Res, 2014 Oct;

352. Whyte G ed., Physiology of Training. Philadelphia: Churchill Livingston Elsevier, 2006

353. Blomstrand E, Eliasson J, Karlsson HKR, Kohnke R, Branched-chain Amino Acids Activate Key Enzymes in Protein Synthesis after Physical Exercise. J Nutr, Jan 2006; 136: 269S-73S

354. Sowers S. A Primer on Branched Chain Amino Acids. Huntington College of Health Sciences, 2009: 1-5

355. Kreher JB, Schwartz JB. Overtraining Syndrome. Sports Health, Mar 2012; 4(2): 128-138.

356. Kreher JB, Schwartz JB. Overtraining Syndrome. Sports Health, Mar 2012; 4(2): 128-138.

357. Suleman A. "Exercise Physiology." emedicine.medscape.com.Medscape. Jul 2013. Web. 10 Oct 2014.

358. Carey DG. Quantifying differences in the 'fat burning" zone and the aerobic zone: implications for training. J Strength Cond Res, 2009; Oct ;23(7): 2090-5.

359. Carey DG. Quantifying differences in the 'fat burning" zone and the aerobic zone: implications for training. J Strength Cond Res, 2009; Oct ;23(7): 2090-5.

360. Westby MD. A health professional's guide to exercise prescription for people with arthritis: a review of aerobic fitness activities. Arthritis Care and Res, 2001; 45(6): 501-511.

361. Hall J, Skevington SM, Maddison PJ, et al. A randomized controlled trial of hydrotherapy in rheumatoid arthritis. Arthritis Care Res, 1996; 9(3): 206-215.

362. Bartels EM, Lund H, Hagen KB, Dagfinrud H, Christensen R, Danneskiold-Sameoe B. Aquatic exercise for the treatment of knee and hip osteoarthritis. Cochrane Database of Systemic Review,. 2007; 4: 1-9.

363. Haskell WL, Lee IM, Pate RR, Powell KE, Blair SN, Franklin BA, Macera CA, Heath GW, Thompson PD, Bauman A. Physical activity and public health: updated recommendation for adults from the American College of Sports Medicine and the American Heart Association. Med Sci Sports Exerc, 2007; 39 (8): 1423-34.

364. US Department of Health and Human Services. Physical Activity Guidelines Advisory Committee Report, 2008[Internet] . Washington (DC): ODPHP Publication No. U0049. 2008[cited 2010 Sep 24].

365. Pollock Ml, Franklin BA, Balady GJ, Chaitman BL, Fleg BA, Fletcher B, Limacher M, Pina IL, Stein RA, Williams M, Bazzarre T. Resistance Exercise in Individuals With and Without Cardiovascular Disease. Circulation, 2000; 101: 828-833.

366. Haskell WL, Lee I-M, Pate RR, et al., Physical activity and public health: Updated recommendations for adults from the American College of Sports Medicine and the American Heart Association. Circulation, 2007; 116 (9): 1081-1093.

367. Ladkowsksi, Edward R. "Are Isometric Exercise a Good Way to Build Strength." Healthy Lifestyle Fitness, Mayo Clinic, 25 Nov 2014. Web . 9 Sept. 2014.

368. Menshikova EV, Ritov VB, Fairfull L, Ferrell RE,Kelley DE, Goodpaster BH. Effects of exercise on mitochondrial content and function in aging human skeletal muscle. Gerontol A Biol Sci Med Sci, June 2006; 61(6): 534-540.

369. Burton DA, Stokes K, Hall GM. Physiologic effects of exercise. Continuing Education in Anesthesia Critical Care & Pain., 2004; 4(6) : 185-188.

370. Clarke PM, Walter SJ, Haven A, Mallon WJ, Heijmans J, Studdert DM. Survival of the fittest:retrospective cohort study of the longevity of Olympic medallists in the modern era. BMJ, 2012;345.

371. Whyte G ed., Physiology of Training. Philadelphia: Churchill Livingston Elsevier, 2006

372. Pool HA, Axford JS. The Effects of Exercise on the Hormonal and Immune Systems in Rheumatoid Arthritis, Rheumatology, 2001, 40: 610-614

373. Cumming DC,Brunsting LA, Strich G, Ries AL, Rebar RW. Reproductive hormone increases in response to acute exercise in men . Medicine and Science in Sports and Exercise, 198618:369-373.,

374. Whyte G ed., Physiology of Training. Philadelphia: Churchill Livingston Elsevier, 2006

375. M Saugy, N Robinson, C Saudan, N Baume, L Avois, and P Mangin, Human growth hormone doping in sport, Br J Sports Med. July 2006; 40(Suppl 1): i35–i39.

376. Despres J-P. Obesity body fat distribution and risk of cardiovascular disease. Circulation, 2012; 125: 130-1313.

377. Klein S. The case of visceral fat – argument for the defense. Journal of Clin Invest, 2004; 113 (11): 1530-1532.

378. Whitworth JA, Williamson PA, Mangos G, Kelly JJ. Cardiovascular Consequences of Cortisol Excess. Vasc Health Risk Manag, Dec 2005;1(4):291-299.

379. Artinian NT, Fletcher GF, Mozaffarian D, Kris –Etherton P, Van Horn L, Lichtenstein AH, Kumanyika S, Kraus WE, Fleg JL, Redeker NS, Meininger JC, Banks J, Stuart –Shor EM, Fletcher BJ, Miller TD, Hughes S, Braun LT, Kopin LA, Berra K, Hayman LL, Ewing LJ, Ades PA, Durstine L, Houston-Miller N, Burke LE. Interventions to promote physical activity and dietary lifestyle changes for cardiovascular risk factor reduction in adults: a scientific statement from the American Heart Association. Circulation, 2010: 122: 406-441.

380. Ross R, Bradshaw wAJ. The future of obesity reduction: beyond weight loss. Nat Rev Endocrinology, 2009: 5: 319-325.

381. Janiszewshi PM, Ross R. Physical activity in the treatment of obesity: beyond weight reduction. Appl Physiol Nutr Metab, 2007; 32: 512-522.

382. Donoho CJ, Weigensberg MJ, Emken BA, Hsu JW, Spriijt-Metz. Stress and abdominal fat: preliminary evidence of ,moderation by the cortisol awakening response in Hispanic peripubertal girls. Obesity, May 2011; 19(5): 946-952.

383. Donoho CJ, Weigensberg MJ, Emken BA,Hsu JW, Spruijt-Metz D. Stress and abdominal fat: preliminary evidence of moderation by the cortisol awakening response in Hispanic peripubertal girls. Obesity, May 2011; 19(5): 946-952.

384. Purnell JQ, Kahn SE, Samuels MH, Brandon D, Loriaux DL, Brunzell JD. Enhanced cortisol production rates, free cortisol, and 11B-HSD-1 expression correlate with visceral fat and insulin resistance in men: effect of weight loss. Am J Physiol Endocrinol Metab, Feb 2009; 296(2): E351-E357.

385. Stanford KI, Middelbeek RJW, Townsend KL, An D, Nygaard EB, Hitchcox KM, Markan KR, Nakano K, Hirshman MF, Tseng Y-H, Goodyear LJ. Brown adipose tissue regulates glucose homeostasis and insulin sensitivity. J Clin Invest, 2013; 123(1): 215-223.

386. Bostrom P, Wu J, Jedrychowski MP, Korde A, Ye L, Lo JC, Rashback KA, Bostrom EA, Choi JH, Long JZ, Kijimura S, Zingaretti MC, Vind BF, Tu H, Cinti S, Hojlund K, Gyqi SP, Spiegelman BM. A PGC1-alpha–dependent myokine that drives brown–fat- like development of white fat and thermogenesis. Nature, Jan 2012; 48(7382): 463-8.

387. Carr DB, Bullen BA, SKrinar GS, Arnold MA, Rosenblatt M, Martin JB, McArthur JW. Physical condition facilitates the exercise–induced secretionof beta–endoprhin and beta–lipotropin in women. N Engl J Med, 1981; 305: 560-563.

388. Boecker H, Sprenger T, Spilker ME, Henriksen G, Koppenhoefer M, Wagner KJ, Valet M, Berthele A, Tolle TR., The runner's high: opiodergic mechanism in the human brain. Cerebral Cortex, 2008 Feb; doi:10.1093/cercor/bhn013.

389. Cooney GM, and Dwan K, Greig CA, Lawlor DA, Rimer J, Waugh FR, Mead GE. Exercise for depression. Cochrane Database of Systematic Reviews, John Wiley & Sons, 12 Sept 2013; Web. 10 Oct 2014.

390. Craft LL, Pernal FM. The benefits of exercise for the clinically depressed. The Primary Care Companion, J Clin Psychiatry, 2004; 6(3): 104-111.

391. Nabkasom C, Miyai N, Sootmongkol A,Junprasert S, Yamamoto H, Arita M, Miyashita K. Effects of physical exercise on depression, neuroendocrine stress hormones and physiological fitness in adolescent females with depressive symptoms. Ment Health Phys Act, Dec 2009; 2(2): 97-99.

392. Agudelo LZ, Femenia T, Orhan F, Porsmyr-Palmertz M, Goiny M,Martinez-Redondo V, Correia JC, Izadi M, Bhat M, Schuppe-Koistinen I, Pettersson AT, Krook A, Barres R, Zierath JR, Erhardt S, Lindskog M, Ruas JL. Skeletal muscle PGC-1alpha 1 modulates kynurenine metabolism and mediates resilience to stress-induced depression. Cell, Sept 2014; 159(1): 33-45.

393. Gomez-Pinilla F, Ying Zhe , Roy R , Molteni R, Edgerton VR. Voluntary exercise induces a BDNF–mediated mechanism that promotes neuroplasticity. Journal of Neurophysiology, 2002; 88(5): 2187-2195.

394. Brown BM, Bourgeat P, Peiffer JJ, Burnham S, Laws SM, Rainey-Smith SR, Bartres-Faz D, Villemagne VL, Taddei K, Rembach A, Bush A, Ellis KA, Macaulay SL, Rowe CC, Ames D, Masters CL, Maruff P, Martins RN. Influence of BDNF Val 66 met on the relationship between physical activity and brain volume. Neurology, 2014 Oct; 8 (15): 1345-52.

395. Erickson KI, Voss MW, Prakash RS. Exercise training increases size of hippocampus and improves memory. PNAS, 2011 Feb;108(7): 3017-3022.

396. Knaepen K, Goekint M, Heyman ME, Meeusen R. Neuroplasticity – exercise–induced response of peripheral brain–derived neurotropic factor. A systematic review of experimental studies in human subjects. Sports Med, Sept; 40(9): 765-801.

397. American Geriatric Society Panel on Exercise and Osteoarthritis. Exercise prescription for older adults with osteoarthritis pain: consensus practice recommendations. A supplement to the AGS Clinical Practice Guidelines on the management of chronic pain in older adults. J Am Geriatr Soc, 2001; 49(6): 808-23.

398. Haskell WL, Lee IM, Pate RR, Powell KE, Blair SN, Franklin BA, Macera CZ, Heath GW, Thompson PD, Bauman A. Physical activity and public health: updated recommendation for adults from the American College of Sports Medicine and the American Heart Association. Med Sci Sports Exerc, 2007; 39 (8): 1423-34.

399. Lee IM, Sesso HD, Paffenbarger RS Jr. Physical activity and coronary heart disease risk in men: does the duration of the exercise episodes predict risk? Circulation, 2000; 102(9): 981-6.

400. Gormley SE, Swain DP, High R, et al., Effect of intensity of aerobic training on VO2 max. Med Sci Sports Exerc, 2008; 40(7): 1335-43.

401. Upadhyay V, Chowdhery A, Bhattacharyya M. Effect of high intensity interval training and slow, continuous training on VO2 max of school going non-athlete males: a comparative study. Br J Sports Med, 2010; 44: 19.

402. Schoenfeld B, Dawes J. High–intensity interval training: applications for general fitness training. Strength & Conditioning Journal, Dec 2009; 31(6): 44-46.

403. Bouri, SZ, Arshadi S. Reaction of resting heart rate and blood pressure to high intensity interval and modern continuous training in coronary artery disease. Br J Sports Med, 2010; 44: i20 doi: 10. 1136bjsm2010.078725.64.

404. Croft L, Bartlett JD, MacLaren DP, Reilly T, Evans L, Mattey DL, Nixon NB, Drust B, Morton JP. High-intensity interval training attenuates the exercise–induced increase in plasma IL-6 in response to acute exercise. Appl Physiol Nutr Metab, 2009; 34

405. Garber CE, Blissmer B, Deschenes MR et al., Quantity and quality of exercise for developing and maintaining cardiorespiratory, musculoskeletal, and neuromotor fitness in apparently healthy adults: guidance for prescribing exercise. Medicine & Science in Sports and Exercise, 2011; DOI : 10.1249/MSS.0b013e318213fefb.

406. Jahnke R, Larkey L, Rogers C , Etnier J, Lin F. A comprehensive review of health benefits of Qigong and tai chi. AM J Health Promot,,Jul –Aug 2010; 24 (6): c1-c25.

407. Jahnke R, Larkey L, Rogers C , Etnier J, Lin F. A comprehensive review of health benefits of Qigong and tai chi. AM J Health Promot, Jul –Aug 2010; 24 (6): c1-c25.

408. Donnelly JE, Blair SN, Jakicic JM,Manore MM, Rankin JW, Smith BK. American College of Sports Medicine: Position Stand: appropriate physical activity intervention strategies for weight loss and prevention of weight regain for adults. Med Sci Sports Exerc, 2009; 41(2): 459-71.

409. Chen H-S, Jap T-S, Chen RL,Lin H-D. A prospective study of glycemic control during holiday time in type 2 diabetic patients. Diabetes Care, 2004 Feb; 27(2): 326-30.

410. Exercise for Strong Bones. National Osteoporosis Foundation. Web. Feb 25 2015.

411. Physical Activity and Cancer. National Cancer Institute. NIH, 22 July 2009; Web. 2014<cancer.gov/cancertopics/causes-prevention/risk-factors/weight-activity/physical-activity-fact-sheet>.

412. Newton RU, Galvao DA. Exercise in prevention and management of cancer. current treatment options in oncology. 2008; 9: 135-146.

413. Braga-Basaria M, Dobs AS, Muller DC,Carducci MA, John M, Egan J, Basaria S. Metabolic syndrome in men with prostate cancer undergoing long-term androgen-deprivation therapy. J Clin Oncol, 2006; 2 (24): 3979-3983.

414. Smith A, Phipps WR, Thomas W. The effects of aerobic exercise on estrogen metabolism in healthy premenopausal women. Cancer Epidemiol Biomarkers Prev, 2013 May; 22(5): 756-764.

415. Anglin RES, Samaan Z, Walter SD. Vitamin D deficiency and depression in adults: systematic review and meta-analysis. BJPsych, 2013 Feb.;A7.DOI:10.1192/bjp.202.2A7.

416. Annweiler C, Schott AM, Allali G, et al., Association of vitamin D deficiency with cognitive impairment in older wormen. Neurology, 2010 Jan.; 74 (1): 27-32.

417. Wang TJ, Pencina MJ, Booth SL, Jaques PF, Ingelsson E, Lanier K, Benjamin EJ, D'Agostino RB, Wolf M, Vasan RS. Vitamin D deficiency and risk of cardiovascular disease. Circulation, 2008; 117: 503-511.

418. Dolgoff-Kaspar R, Baldwin A, Johnson MS. Effect of laughter yoga on mood and heart rate variability in patients awaiting organ transplantation: a pilot study. Altern Ther Health Med, 2012 Sep- Oct; 18(5): 61-6.

419. Yazdani, M, Esmaeilzadeh M, Pahlavanzadeh S, Khaledi F. The effects of laughter yoga on general health among nursing students. Iran J Nurs Midwifery Res, 2014 Jan; 19(1); 36-40.

GLOSSARY

CHAPTER 1:

CONSTIPATION: a condition where there is difficulty emptying the bowels often due to dehydration; associated with harden stools

MULTIPLE SCLEROSIS: an autoimmune illness where the immune system attacks the protective covering of nerves

RHEUMATOID ARTHRITIS: an autoimmune illness where the immune system attacks the joints

INFLAMMATORY BOWEL DISEASE: chronic inflammation of part or all of the digestive tract; can be associated with abdominal pain, bloody diarrhea and joint pain

INFLAMMATION: The presence of an activated immune system which produces chemicals when there are injuries, infection, damaged cells, or irritants in the body.

BODY MASS INDEX: Height to weight ratio that categorize people as normal size, overweight and obese. Obesity is associated with development of chronic disease.

BODY COMPOSITION: a calculation of the percentage of fat, muscle, bone, and water in a human

PERCENTAGE BODY FAT: The amount of fat in our bodies.

C-REACTIVE PROTEIN: a blood test which is used to gauge and monitor inflammation. It is nonspecific and could suggest inflammation anywhere in the body.

CARDIAC C-REACTIVE PROTEIN: More specific measure to inflammation in the heart

ERYTHROCYTE SEDIMENTATION RATE: a nonspecific blood test which is used to monitor inflammation

HOMEOSTASIS: The tendency of the body to create internal stability and equilibrium, despite stressors. It is the body's need to have balance

PHYTONUTRIENTS: chemicals that are in plants, fruits and vegetables which assist with disease prevention and maintaining health

AMINO ACIDS: Building blocks of protein

TOXINS: Substances which can be poisonous to our body.

DETOXIFICATION: removal of substances which can be poisonous to our body

CHAPTER 2:

HDL: a type of cholesterol which is favorable

LDL: a subtype of cholesterol which is implicated in forming plaque

SATURATED FAT: a type of fat that has no double bonds, found in animal fats and many oils

HYDROGENATED OILS: Process in which a hydrogen bond is added to a liquid phase of oil to turn it into a solid; increases shelf life of a product

OXIDATIVE STRESS: Stress on the body that triggers formation of toxic chemicals, free radicals

CHAPTER 3:

WORLD HEALTH ORGANIZATION: Health arm of the United Nations which focuses on international public health.

TERTIARY CARE HOSPITAL: a hospital which is designated as a center of excellence and offers specialty and high acuity services

INSOMNIA: the symptom of the inability to sleep

IRRITABLE BOWEL SYNDROME: a chronic intestinal disorder which manifests as a symptom complex: cramping, bloating, constipation or diarrhea

ELEMENTARY PREVENTION: tools that we use to prevent the onset of illness

FUNCTIONAL MEDICINE: type of medicine which focuses on a multi-system approach to disease. It looks at the interactions of the environment and the gastrointestinal, endocrine, and immune systems

CARBOHYDRATES: a type of nutrient found in food which is important for energy production and forms into glucose

GENETICALLY MODIFIED (GMO): a food or crop which has genetic material that has been artificially altered

CHAPTER 4:

EUSTRESS: a term coined by Dr. Hans Seyle; the beneficial effects to the mind and body of stress

DISTRESS: the detrimental effects to the mind and body from stress

GENERAL ADAPTATION SYNDROME: The physiologic process of how the body responds to a new stress.

AUTONOMIC NERVOUS SYSTEM: a part of the nervous system which influences the function of internal organs.

SYMPATHETIC NERVOUS SYSTEM: one division of the autonomic nervous system which regulates the body's fight or flight response in times of stress and danger

PARASYMPATHETIC NERVOUS SYSTEM: one division of the autonomic nervous system which regulates the body's rest and digest system in times of calm and relaxation

NEUROTRANSMITTERS: chemicals which transmit the signals across nerve cells

EPINEPHRINE: a hormone released by the adrenal gland during a stress response which raises the heart rate and blood pressure

NOREPINEPHRINE: a hormone released by the adrenal gland during a stress response which raises the heart rate and blood pressure

IMMUNE SYSTEM: the system in the body which works to protect the body from disease; system that fights against infections and other abnormal cells

ENDOCRINE: a system in the body which produces hormones which regulate many functions of the body such as metabolism, growth and development, reproduction, sexual function , sleep and mood.

CARDIOVASCULAR SYSTEM: a system in the body which involves the heart and blood vessels

CORTISOL: a hormone secreted by the adrenal gland released in response to stress

GLYCOGENOLYSIS: the breakdown of glycogen into glucose

LIPOLYSIS: the breakdown of fats and lipids

MACROPHAGES: type of white cells which work on getting rid of damaged cells and fighting infections

NATURAL KILLER CELLS: type of white cells which respond to viral infections and tumor cells

FREE RADICALS: Harmful toxins triggered by stress

COGNITION: the process of acquiring knowledge through thought

GENES: Basic unit of heredity; made up of DNA; they make us who we are.

CHROMOSOMES: structures inside the nucleus of a cell which house the DNA

TELOMERES: the region at the ends of a chromosome which protects it from deterioration

COLLAGEN: is the structural protein in the space outside cells which offers strength and structure to our bodies

CHAPTER 5:

PRE-DIABETES: mild elevations in blood glucose

DIABETES: An illness which is categorized by difficulty processing glucose. There are different types which are based on if the insulin is being generated by the pancreas. The diagnosis is made if the fasting glucose is over 126 more than two checks or if the HBA1c is over 6.5 g/dL.

CARDIOVASCULAR DISEASE/HEART DISEASE: class of illness which involves the heart and blood vessels

STROKE: an illness where poor blood flow to the brain causes injury and even the death of the brain cells.

OVERWEIGHT: A term used to define excess weight. It is defined by a BMI between 25-29.9 kg/m2

OBESITY: A term used to define excess weight. It is defined by a BMI 30 kg/m2 or higher.

ALZHEIMER'S DISEASE: A form of memory loss which is the most common form of dementia. It is characterized by amyloid plaques

COLON CANCER: A type of cancer which affects the large intestine or rectum.

PANCREATIC CANCER: A type of cancer which affects the pancreas.

AUTOIMMUNE DISEASE: A class of illness which involves the over activation of the immune system forcing the body to attack its own tissues.

OSTEOARTHRITIS: A type of degenerative arthritis mostly due to wear and tear.

INSULIN RESISTANCE (IR): Insulin is a hormone which is required for the cells to take up glucose. IR is a condition where the cells of the body become increasingly resistant to the effects of insulin.

HORMONES: Proteins in the blood which travel from one site to another to cause changes.

RECEPTORS: a region on a cell membrane which responds to a particular hormone or substance

PLAQUE: a substance made up of fat, cholesterol, calcium and inflammatory cells found in the blood. Over time, it can harden and block flow of oxygen rich blood.

CORONARY ARTERIES: the blood vessels which supply the heart muscle

ENDOTHELIUM: single cell layer which lines the interior surface of the blood vessels

ENDOTHELIUM DYSFUNCTION: a pathologic state of the single cell layer of the lining of the blood vessels which prevents the blood vessel from dilating

ATHEROSCLEROSIS: the build-up of plaque in and on artery walls

STATINS: medications to lower cholesterol which block a pathway that forms cholesterol in the liver

MYELIN SHEATHS: the protective covering of nerves including brain and spinal cord. It allows electrical impulses to transmit efficiently along nerves

NERVE CONDUCTION: the movement of an electrical impulse along a nerve

ACANTHOSIS NIGRICANS: black or brown discoloration of the skin which is found in skin folds such as armpits, neck, and groin.

HYPERTENSION: An illness which a person has persistently elevated blood pressure

CHAPTER 6:

MICROBIOME: the collective genome of the microorganisms which share our body

MICROBIOTA: the collective community of microorganisms which share our body

CLOSTRIDIUM DIFFICILE COLITIS (C. DIFF): an inflammatory illness of the large intestine secondary to a bacteria called Clostridium Difficile

MICROORGANISMS: a living organism which is single celled and is microscopic.

GENOME: complete set of DNA of an organism

AMINO ACIDS: building blocks of protein

TYPE I DIABETES: A type of disorder of glucose metabolism where the pancreas cannot generate insulin.

GUT-BRAIN AXIS: The connection which is based on the biochemical signaling between the nervous system (brain) and the gastrointestinal tract (gut)

SUBCONSCIOUS: part of the mind of a person which is not fully aware but can influence actions and feelings

VAGUS NERVE: A nerve that spreads into the gastrointestinal tract and the heart and is a large component of the parasympathetic nervous system

TRYPTOPHAN: is an amino acid which is a precursor to serotonin. It is considered an essential amino acid since your body can not make it, it must be consumed

SEROTONIN: a biochemical regulator or neurotransmitter which is thought to regulate mood. It is predominantly found in the GI tract.

GERM-FREE HOST: usually a rat or mouse which has been eradicated of all its microbiota

NEURODEGENERATIVE DISORDER: an illness which causes progressive deterioration of the nervous system

NEUROCOGNITIVE DISORDER: an illness which causes deterioration of the ability to formulate new knowledge and access and process existing knowledge

AUTISM: an illness which is characterized by difficulties in social interactions, with verbal and nonverbal communication and notable for repetitive behavior

T CELL: A type of white blood cell which is part of the immune system; responsible for fighting infection

INTESTINAL MUCOSA: The cells which are in contact with the open space or lumen of the digestive tract. It comes in direct contact with digested food

EPITHELIAL BARRIER: the layer of the colon that is in contact with the food and the external environment

HYGIENE HYPOTHESIS: a theory which states that a decreased early exposure to infectious agents, good microorganisms and parasites increases risk to allergenic disease by suppressing the natural development of our immune system

SHORT CHAIN FATTY ACIDS: end products of fermentation of fiber by anaerobic bacteria of the intestinal lining which have shown to exert multiple beneficial effects

BACTEROIDES: bacteria found in the gut

FIRMICUTES: bacteria found in the gut

SHIGELLA: a bacteria which has been implicated with causing gastrointestinal illness like dysentery

E COLI: gram negative bacteria which is part of normal gut flora

DYSBIOSIS: a condition where the bacterial flora is not in balance.

LEPTIN: a hormone made by fat cells which regulate hunger and help us feel full.

MACROPHAGES: cells of the immune system which are associated with defense against foreign cells and start plaque formation

TNF-: a substance released by the immune system in response to insult

IL-1: a substance released by the immune system in response to insult

IL-6: a substance released by the immune system in response to insult

CHEMOKINES: are chemicals which attract white cells when inflammation is present

NITRIC OXIDE (NO): gas which dilates the blood vessels

ARACHIDONIC ACID DERIVATIVES: thromboxane A2, prostaglandins E2 and F1 , substances that have inflammatory and regenerative properties

TNF-ALPHA: a substance released by the immune system in response to insult

LIPOPOLYSACCHARIDE: molecules found on the outer membrane of certain types of bacteria and can elicit a strong immune response

CYTOKINES: small proteins involved with cell signaling

ATHEROGENESIS: The formation of plaque

PHOSPHATIDYL CHOLINE: a lipid found on the membrane of cells

TRIMETHYLAMINE-N-OXIDE (TMAO): a substance which is formed by bacteria in our gut which promotes the formation of plaque in our blood vessels

INTESTINAL PERMEABILITY: Weakening of the bowel wall

CELIAC DISEASE: a genetically predisposing autoimmune disease which is characterized by damage to the lining of the small intestine due to a severe reaction to gluten

MALABSORPTION: characterized by a difficulty in absorption of nutrients from food

OCCLUDIN: a protein is responsible for the tight junctions in the cells that line the digestive tract

ZONULIN: a protein which affects the permeability of the tight junctions between cells that line the digestive tract

PROBIOTICS: microorganisms which are ingested

RESISTANT STARCHES: type of dietary fiber naturally found in carbohydrate foods which can help grow the good bacteria in our digestive tract

CHAPTER 7:

CARDIAC CATHETERIZATION: a procedure which is done where a small tube is placed in a blood vessel. A dye is placed the catheter to help visualize blockages in the vessels surrounding the heart.

DIVERTICULOSIS: A medical condition characterized by the presence of small pouches in the large intestine

LIPOPOLYSACCHARIDE: molecules found on the outer membrane of certain types of bacteria and can elicit a strong immune response

ENDOTHELIAL DYSFUNCTION: a pathologic state of the single cell layer of the lining of the blood vessels which prevents the blood vessel from dilating

HETEROCYCLIC AMINES: compounds which are created when cooking foods at high temperature

CARCINOGENS: any substance or compound which can be directly involved with causing cancer

TMAO: Trimethylamine N-oxide: a substance which is formed by bacteria in our gut which promotes the formation of plaque in our blood vessels

POLYCYCLIC AROMATIC HYDROCARBONS: organic compounds which are formed when there is insufficient oxygen; often found when foods are cooked at high temperatures and thought to be carcinogenic

PASTEURIZATION: a process of heating which is intended to reduce the number of microorganisms in the foods

LUPUS: short for Systemic Lupus Erythematosus which is an autoimmune disease which can affect skin, joints and organs in the body

VITILIGO: a chronic skin condition where the portions of the body lose skin pigment

GENE TRANSCRIPTION FACTORS: proteins which allow for the reading of genes and generating the proteins which they code for

TYPE I DIABETES: High blood sugars due to an autoimmune process where the body attacks the insulin forming cells

TYPE II DIABETES: high blood sugars due to the resistance of the body to the actions of insulin

CASEIN: the protein found in milk and dairy products

GALACTOSE: the sugar which is found in milk and dairy products

LACTOSE: sugar made from galactose and glucose and primarily found in milk and dairy products

GLUCOSE: an umbrella term for sugar; used as energy for our cells; high levels are associated with diabetes

PROTEIN: large molecules which are composed of amino acids

PRESERVATIVE: a substance which is added to food and beverages to help prevent its decomposition by growth of microbial or by chemical changes

CALORIE DENSITY: calories per density of food; higher caloric density have more calories in a smaller space

TRANS-FATS: chemically engineered fats which are used to make oils more solid at room temperature; increases shelf life

AMERICAN ACADEMY OF ENVIRONMENTAL MEDICINE: an international organization which represents physicians who specialize in looking at the interactions of environment and its impact on health

CHAPTER 8:

PHYTONUTRIENTS: chemicals in plants, fruits and vegetables which protect them from plant from environmental and infectious agents but also have health promoting properties such as high content of antioxidants and anti-inflammatory properties.

PLANT STEROLS: naturally occurring substances found in grains, vegetables, fruits, legumes, nuts and seeds which have cholesterol lowering properties

CAROTENOIDS: a yellow, orange or red pigment found in plants, fruits and vegetables which offer antioxidant benefits to cells.

FLAVONOIDS: a plant based compound found in fruits and vegetables which offer antioxidant benefits. Common foods high in flavonoids are onions, parsley, blueberries, bananas, dark chocolate and red wine.

RESVERATROL: a natural chemical produced in plants in response to an injury or when the plant is under attack by a fungus or bacteria. Found in high levels in skin of grapes.

PHYTOESTROGENS: plant derived natural substances which have structural similarity to estrogen made by the ovaries and can bind to estrogen receptors and can cause estrogen or antiestrogen effects

ANTI-OXIDANTS: substances that may prevent or delay types of cell damage

ALPHA LINOLEIC ACID: is a fatty acid which is essential for health and cannot be made by the body so it must be consumed through diet; a precursor to formation of omega 3 fatty acids

LINOLEIC ACID: a fatty acid which is essential for health and cannot be made by the body so it must be consumed through the diet; part of the omega 6 fatty acid chain.

FRUCTOSE: a simple sugar when combined with glucose forms sucrose

MACULAR DEGENERATION: a medical illness which is associated with damage to the retina of the eye and can cause blindness and visual impairment in adults

GLYCEMIC INDEX: numerical index from 0 to 100 which ranks carbohydrates by the rate of their conversion to glucose in the body; higher glycemic index converts more easily to glucose.

SHORT CHAIN FATTY ACIDS: acids which are beneficial to the cells of the gut which are formed when foods are digested by bacteria in the gut

MYOCARDIAL INFARCTION: plaque rupture in the heart that causes damage to the heart muscle due to lack of blood supply

FERMENTATION: metabolic process which involves the conversion of sugar to gases, alcohol or acids

PROBIOTICS: ingested microorganisms aimed to replenish gut flora

KETOSIS: a metabolic process where there is low carbohydrate volume and energy production has to shift to primarily from fat sources

CHAPTER 9:

UNSATURATED FATS: a fatty acid or fat which there is one or more double bond, found in vegetable oils, avocados and nuts

MONOUNSATURATED FATS: a fatty acid or fat which there is one double bond, often found in olive oil

POLYUNSATURATED FATS: a fatty acid or fat which there is more than one double bond, found in many vegetable oils

OMEGA 3 FATTY ACIDS: polyunsaturated fats that are broken into eicosapentaenoic acids (EPA) and docosahexaenoic acids (DHA); found in walnuts, chia and flax seeds

ESSENTIAL FATTY ACIDS: fats which cannot be generated from the body and must be taken in through the diet. Examples are linoleic and alpha linoleic acid.

ATHEROSCLEROSIS: A medical condition where is generation of plaque in the arteries

CORONARY HEART DISEASE: the most common type of heart disease which occurs when the arteries supplying blood to the heart become narrowed and hardened

TRIGLYCERIDES: a type of fat which is found in the blood and where high levels are thought to be a risk factor for heart disease

PLATELET AGGREGATION: the act of the platelet cells sticking together to help stop bleeding and form a clot

CALORIE DENSITY: calories per density of food; higher caloric density foods have more calories in a smaller space

ALZHEIMER'S DISEASE: the most common type of dementia which is categorized by the presence of beta amyloid plaques and tangles

LIGNANS: chemical compound found in plants which have antioxidant effects

TRYPTOPHAN: an amino acid which is the precursor to serotonin

CHAPTER 10:

NEUROPROTECTIVE: something which has the ability to protect brain, spinal cord and nerves

ATHEROSCLEROTIC PLAQUE: plaque in the blood vessel (artery) walls

SAPONINS: chemical compounds found in plants which are thought to protect the plant against microbes and fungi

CHAPTER 11:

METABOLISM: process by which there is conversion of food into energy often referred to in terms of weight management

CHAPTER 12:

ADHD: attention deficit hyperactivity disorder; a medical condition characterized by difficulty staying focused, paying attention, controlling behavior and hyperactivity

CIRCADIAN RHYTHM: a cycle of 24 hours which can affect physical, mental and behavioral changes

ADENOSINE: a neurotransmitter in the brain which can promote sleep and suppress arousal.

MELATONIN: a hormone which promotes sleep

NATIONAL SLEEP FOUNDATION: an organization which has resources for sleep research and education regarding sleep disorders

REM: Rapid Eye Movement- a stage of sleep characterized by rapid eye movements; considered the dream state

SLEEP LATENCY: the amount of time it takes from lying down to sleep till the onset of sleep

SLEEP FRAGMENTATION: the disturbance in sleep which is notable for interruption of the sleep stages

NEURODEGENERATIVE CONDITIONS: a broad term for illnesses which primarily affect the neurons in the brain

PARKINSON'S DISEASE: a medical illness which is characterized by a movement disorder associated with a resting tremor

DEMENTIA: a general term which implies a decline in mental function which is severe enough to impact daily life

BENIGN PROSTATIC HYPERTROPHY: a medical condition which is characterized by the growth in size of the prostate gland from a non-cancerous cause; associated with decreased urination

SLEEP APNEA: a medical condition characterized by disruption of sleep due to low oxygen levels in the brain

GLUTATHIONE: a substance made naturally in the liver which is an antioxidant

HIV: Human Immunodeficiency Virus; causes marked suppression of the immune system

PSYCHOMOTOR PERFORMANCE: coordination of motor activity with a sensory or cognitive process

GHRELIN: a hormone which has a role in triggering appetite

LEPTIN: a hormone which has a role in triggering satiety

HIPPOCAMPUS: a; part of the brain which has a major role in memory

NONSENSE SYLLABLES: syllables which have no meaning used in songs or used in memory, experiments or tests

MAMMILLARY BODIES: part of the brain that is involved in recognitional memory; such as remembering that you had seen someone before

HYPOXIA/HYPOXIC: a deficiency in the oxygen amount which reaches the tissues

ISCHEMIA/ISCHEMIC: damage to an organ or part of the body when there is a low flow of blood or oxygen

CYTOKINES: small proteins involved with cell signaling

PHOTOSENSITIVE RETINAL GANGLION CELLS: a type of nerve cell in the retina of the eye which signal the presence of light

BETA BRAIN WAVES: EEG patterns found to represent activity of brain when it is alert, engaged in problem solving, focused activity or judgement decision making

PINEAL GLAND: a small endocrine gland in the brain which secretes melatonin

INTERSTITIAL SPACE: the space between cells of a tissue which are fluid filled

CEREBROSPINAL FLUID: clear fluid found in the brain and the spine which acts as a protective cushion for the brain and spinal cord

AMYLOID B: amyloid beta which are proteins that are implicated in the formation of Alzheimer's disease

NEUROTOXINS: any chemical or substance which can cause damage to a nerve cell

SYMPATHETIC OVERDRIVE: the state of having a persistent activation to a stress response

CHAPTER 13:

PRANAYAMA BREATHING: formal practice of control and extension of breath

ASANAS: physical aspect of yoga which relates to benefits from the postures

ISOMETRIC: type of strength training in which the joint angle does not change.

ISOTONIC: a type of exercise where the muscle tone is kept constant tension during the movement. Examples are squats, push –ups, and pull ups.

PREFRONTAL CORTEX: an area of the brain in the frontal lobe which implicated in planning complex cognitive behavior, personality expression and decision making

AUDITORY LEARNING: the act of learning new material through sound and speech

ATROPHY: a tissue or organ which wastes away due to degeneration of the cells

MINDFULNESS: a meditative state where the focus of attention is on the present moment

DHEA: a hormone secreted by the adrenal gland

ADIPONECTIN: a hormone produced and secreted by fat cells which regulate metabolism of glucose and fats

POLYCYSTIC OVARY DISEASE: a medical condition characterized by the presence of insulin resistance associated with menstrual irregularities, infertility, abnormal glucose and excessive hair growth in women

YOGA NIDHRA: a form of guided meditation which helps with relaxation

SIVASANA: a pose in yoga for total relaxation; also called the corpse pose.

COPD: Chronic Obstructive Pulmonary Disease- a medical illness characterized by blocked airflow and difficulty breathing

ATP: Adenosine Triphosphate: the end product in many cellular reactions which serves as an energy source

NF-KAPPA B: a protein complex which controls the transcription of DNA, cytokine production and survival of the cell; plays a key role in modulating the immune response in times of stress.

CHAPTER 14:

METABOLIC EQUIVALENT-MET: a physiologic measure which expresses the energy cost of physical activities

CALORIE/KILOCALORIE: Terms are often used interchangeably; one calorie is the energy required to raise the temperature of 1 gram of water by 1 degree Celsius. It is used frequently to identify the energy obtained by intake of food. 1000 calories equal 1 kilocalorie

ANAEROBIC: In exercise, it is when the exercise is intense where oxygen demands cannot be kept up and enough to trigger the formation of lactic acid

AEROBIC: exercise which is intended to improve the efficiency of the cardiovascular system of the body in absorbing and transporting oxygen

METABOLIC FITNESS: the benefits which occur when muscles become more efficient at utilizing their resources. Indirectly can be measured by glucose tolerance and lipid profiles

LACTIC ACID: normal byproduct of anaerobic muscle metabolism which is associated with discomfort and soreness

ADRENALINE: also known as epinephrine; a neurotransmitter which is released by the adrenal gland in response to stress

NITRIC OXIDE: a gas which dilates the blood vessels

OVERREACHING SYNDROME: a compilation of symptoms which occurs when the balance between training and recovery is not proportionate and usually lasts 2 weeks

OVERTRAINING: training is significantly outweighed by recovery; causes a compilation of symptoms which can last weeks to months

RESPIRATORY RATE: breathing rate per minute

VO2 MAX: maximum rate of oxygen uptake as measured during incremental exercise

MAXIMUM PREDICTED HEART RATE (MPHR): 220-age. Achieving 85% MPHR is associated with better cardiovascular outcomes

OSTEOARTHRITIS: a degenerative form of arthritis notable for breakdown due to wear and tear

RESISTANCE EXERCISE: exercise which causes a muscle to contract against external resistance

ISOTONIC EXERCISE: a type of exercise where the joint angle and muscle length change such as with squats

ISOMETRIC EXERCISE: a type of exercise where the joint angle and the muscle length do not change such as with planks

STROKE VOLUME: the amount of blood pumped out of the heart with each contraction

MITOCHONDRIA: a vital part of cells and tissues where energy production occurs

HYPERTROPHY: enlargement of a tissue or organ

ANABOLIC HORMONES: hormones which are primarily in charge of building the body

SUBCUTANEOUS FAT: the fat which is under the skin

VISCERAL FAT: fat which surrounds organs in the abdominal cavity

POSITRON EMISSION TOMOGRAPHY: type of imaging test using radioactive dye that allows us to detect disease in the body

ENDORPHINS: naturally produced by the brain; these peptides have opiate like activities and can reduce pain naturally

PGC–1 ALPHA 1 PROTEIN: induced by skeletal muscle by exercise and endurance that has a protective effect against depression

KYNURENINE: a metabolite of the amino acid L-tryptophan; has a role in inflammation

BRAIN DERIVED NEUROTROPIC FACTOR (BDNF): a protein which has a role in supporting survival of existing neurons and is vital to learning and memory

NEUROPLASTICITY: the ability to of neural pathways to change due to changes in behavior, environment, thinking, emotions, injury and disease.

IL-6: cytokine which has a strong role in stimulating an inflammatory response during infections and trauma

TNF-ALPHA: a cell signaling protein which is involved in the acute phase reaction and recruits cells that invoke a response to a stress, inflammation and infections.

COLORECTAL CANCER: often an umbrella term used for cancer of the colon

ADIPOSITY: a word used to describe the quantity of fat tissue

ENDOMETRIAL: pertaining to the lining of the uterus

ACKNOWLEDGMENTS

WE WOULD LIKE TO ACKNOWLEDGE a few people without whom, this book would not have been possible. First we want to thank Dr. Parthiv Mahadevia and Mr. Robert Snodgrass who have helped read and reread and reread the chapters of the book. We would also like to thank Mona Shroff and Kosha Dalal for helping with edits and Anjali Shroff for helping us by taking great food photos. We would like to thank Shilpa Johnson for giving us innovative recipes. We would like to thank Philip Hicks who helped us personally to get stronger and helped us put together exercises for all ages. We would like to also thank two very influential people. Karen Fick is an amazing person and who helped Dr. Aggarwal start on her journey to healing. Dr. A will always be thankful to her for that. We also want to thank Bob Lascaro who has been an amazing designer, advisor and guide with putting this book together and without whom, none of this would have been possible.